PRAISE FOR
THE FUTURE OF NUTRITION

"Just finished this book and can't stop talking about it to whomever will listen to me. It is fantastic. Colin Campbell's latest masterpiece on whole food, plant-based (WFPB) nutrition is a must read for anybody interested in understanding health, cancer, and how a proven lifestyle has become so controversial. Campbell sets the tone for how WFPB can guide us toward optimal living."

—David Feinberg, MD, head of Google Health

"Dr. Campbell serves up a sweeping historical survey of the literature on diet and health, brilliantly exploring the institutional biases that have long confused consumers and subverted the science as to the power of evidence-based nutrition to prevent and treat disease. Couldn't put the book down!"

—Michael Greger, MD, bestselling author of *How Not to Die*

"T. Colin Campbell is legendary when it comes to nutrition. His six decades of scientific work and advocacy changed the world's understanding of how what we eat can cause or prevent cancer. In *The Future of Nutrition*, Campbell prophesizes a healthier planet populated by healthier people eating a whole food, plant-based diet. To get us there, Campbell reveals a long-standing opponent: a confrontational nutrition establishment that must evolve to embrace modern science and move beyond its outdated thinking. Through his eyes and acerbic wit, we learn about the fascinating and, at times, outrageous academic, political, and industrial intrigue that has tripped up efforts to improve our nation's diet for more than one hundred years. Campbell delivers decisive directions on what needs to be done to move our communities towards a healthier, evidence-based way of eating. *The Future of Nutrition* is Campbell's magnum opus and will leave you rethinking how you discuss healthy eating, what you hear about dietary guidelines, and what's in your next bite. This is a must read for everyone who is serious about nutrition and wants a unique behind-the-scenes understanding of a foe-ridden field through the eyes of a pioneer."

—William W. Li, MD, *New York Times* bestselling author of *Eat to Beat Disease* and president and medical director of the Angiogenesis Foundation

"Dr. Campbell, the pioneering researcher whose earlier published findings in *The China Study* on the benefits of plant-based versus animal-based foods 'fired the shot heard round the world,' does it again in *The Future of Nutrition*. This book is a must-read for many reasons, the main one being that our health and our lives depend on us acting on the tipping point evidence that Dr. Campbell provides. He exposes the bribery and graft that occurs hidden from us and uses our own tax dollars to deliberately mislead us, the American public. He tells it like it was and, unfortunately, how it still is. It is obvious that Dr. Campbell's towering intellect, (plus his wry humor), and dedication to dig into the archives and expose the purposely hidden information and corruption related to the power of food—and money. He reveals this by naming names complete with citations. We are in the midst of a human-caused mass extinction which can be reversed by following the logical steps of halting the damage being done to our environment. All is not lost YET, but only if enough of us implement the calls to action that Dr. Campbell outlines that will help us recognize where we are going wrong, how we can reverse course, stop fighting Nature and get back in tune with her. I'll add my call to action: Get as many others to read this book as you can because we must act now."

—**Ruth Heidrich, PhD, WFPB Ironman triathlete and author of** *A Race For Life* **and** *Senior Fitness*

"As a cellist, I know that true music is much more than the parts. An inexplicable magic occurs when there is harmony between the physical and spiritual. After reading this book, the truth of wholism and living at one with nature became much more than well documented science. Everything came together as a whole and made music. This book had a huge impact on me. I think it will change many lives for the better."

—**Daniel Domb, cello soloist with the New York Philharmonic, Boston Pops, Chicago Symphony, National Symphony, Cleveland Orchestra, and The Three Tenors, and recitalist at Carnegie Hall, Concertgebouw, and Wigmore Hall**

"Dr. Colin Campbell, the quintessential scientist and nutrition researcher, steps us through the radical controversy and confusion surrounding nutrition and cancer research. Dr. Campbell eloquently unpacks the science of nutrition and its far-reaching potential to prevent, reverse, and treat chronic disease. *The Future of Nutrition* is a critical read for those seeking to improve their health, their community, and the planet!"

—**Michael C. Hollie, MD, FACLM, speaker for Dinner with the Doctor**

"In *The Future of Nutrition*, Dr. Colin Campbell delivers yet another masterpiece! *The Future of Nutrition* elucidates the many intricate nuances between the complex interfaces of the nutritional and medical sciences. Pertinent historical narratives form an important backdrop to this insightful discussion. Dr. Campbell walks us through much of the salient scientific evidence that has clearly shown the benefits of a whole food plant-based diet against chronic illnesses. At the time of this writing, the United States and most of the world is in the midst of a viral pandemic that has exposed our general poor health and disrupted our way of living. The time has come for the medical community to acknowledge the indisputable evidence of the power of plant-based nutrition in removing the grip that chronic illness has on our lives. This book is a *must read* for physicians, medical scientists, and the general public."

—Baxter Montgomery, MD, FACC, Clinical Assistant Professor of Medicine, Division of Cardiology/Cardiac Electrophysiology, University of Texas Health Science Center, Houston

"Colin Campbell is a scientist specializing in nutrition. So what? Well, he also happens to be one of the world's leading experts in his field, but there's more. As he explains in this book, genuine nutritional scientists are surprisingly rare nowadays, because the entire edifice of food science is thoroughly corrupt, from top to bottom. The main reason for this is the Western world's addiction to meat. The signs are all there: like any other drug addict, the Western nutritional establishment have woven a web of lies over centuries to rationalise their behaviour, which has deeply harmful effects on others. It's a major factor contributing to the current global environmental crisis, it's ruining our health and our economies, and it's the reason why so many animals—at least 70 billion land animals per year—endure short, tortured lives in factory farms. Tellingly, when Campbell was once giving a presentation about food, he received a self-pitying, emotional complaint from a fellow food researcher, an MIT professor no less: 'Colin, you're talking about good food. Please don't take it away from us!' But Campbell is a genuine food scientist, and it's his job to hold up the mirror of truth to the ugly face of our meat addiction. In this, his latest book, he lays out the basic facts, clearly and understandably. Will it be enough to encourage people to 'go cold turkey about cold turkey and other meats'? That remains to be seen; he can do no more."

—Gordon Mackenzie, first-class degree in philosophy from Durham University (UK), English teacher in eastern Europe, and translator in France and Belgium

"Buckle up for an incredible ride! The Future of Nutrition gives the reader an unvarnished front row view of the forces that have had profound influence, for better or for worse, on the food we literally place at the end of our forks. Controversy, vested interests, ostracism, and bias—the stuff typically reserved for soap operas—took center stage in shaping something much more fundamental: the food we eat. Dr. Campbell, an ethical pillar with a seat at the table, has been immersed in this space for decades. Unapologetically upending orthodoxy and prevailing norms, this incredible adventure concludes with powerful calls to action."

**—Robert Ostfeld, MD, MSc, FACC, professor of medicine and
director of preventive cardiology for the Montefiore Health System**

"Since 1960, Dr. Campbell's work has cast an ever-brightening light into the darkness of nutritional science—and his sixty-year journey is documented in this meticulously referenced book. Largely based on knowledge garnered from him on this crucial topic, it ultimately became obvious to me that if we cannot take the animal out of the equation when it comes to feeding ourselves, we will never learn to live in harmony with nature—thereby placing the future of our civilization (and our species) in serious jeopardy. As such, if we Homo sapiens somehow manage to save ourselves from extinction—much of the credit should go to T. Colin Campbell."

**—J. Morris Hicks, author of *Outcry*, *Healthy Eating,
Healthy World* and the *4Leaf Guide to Vibrant Health***

"Reflux, a too common medical malady, creates significant suffering and concern for millions. Like most chronic diseases, reflux is diet based. Diet alone can prevent and reverse symptoms and prevent complications, including esophageal cancer. The problem is with misinformation and lack of information much like the myriad diseases discussed in this book. In *The Future of Nutrition*, Dr. T. Colin Campbell synthesizes a comprehensive overview of the difficulty in disseminating nutritional information to the public in a manner that they can listen, hear, and change. His personal experience and knowledge of the influence of industry and politics in the realm of nutrition provides many answers as to why the science of nutrition lags behind the adoption of dietary change in preventing and reversing chronic disease."

**—Craig H. Zalvan, MD, FACS, Chief of Otolaryngology and
Medical Director, The Institute for Voice and Swallowing Disorders
at Phelps Hospital, Professor of Otolaryngology at the Donald and
Barbara Zucker School of Medicine at Hofstra/Northwell**

"In detailing his 45 years of experience as a student, researcher, and professor at Cornell University, Dr. Campbell reveals his experience navigating the complex political landscape of academia, wherein universities all too often exclude life-saving information from curricula to protect their bottom lines. Over the course of my Cornell education, I was repeatedly confronted with the fundamental truth that academia is beholden to outdated traditions, dogma, and stakeholders which influence and filter information taught by credible institutions. The context provided by Dr. Campbell allows students of all disciplines to think critically about the information they consume, with recognition that industry-led parties stand to benefit from the dissemination of certain forms of knowledge."

—**Chloe Cabrera, Cornell University, BS 2019,**
Cornell University (graduate studies, exp 2021)

"In *The Future of Nutrition*, Dr. Campbell draws upon his six decades of pioneering scientific research, navigating a complicated history of the impact of powerful institutions on food, health, and ultimately disease in our society. Opening the curtain, he sheds light on the growing cancer of corporate influence in academia, which has metastasized throughout our societal system. As a millennial and passionate plant-based educator, there is an increasing urgency to fight for nutrition justice now and for generations to come. Dr. Campbell's research about how food can heal, paves the way."

—**Ella Stephens, Cornell University, BS 2017 (Nutritional Sciences),**
Wageningen University, Netherlands (graduate studies)

"Dr. Campbell has shed light on the lack of integrity in the medical and nutrition fields, arguing that individual shortcomings reflect a systemic, societal issue; when faced with solutions benefiting society in the long term, those in power actively choose to make capital and individualistic gains for the short term. As a graduate of Cornell University's Nutrition program, the evidence presented in this book both affirmed my undergraduate experiences and shocked my understanding of the healthcare fields. This book not only presents the truths behind the prevailing ideas and confusions surrounding nutrition and medicine but unmasks the ultimate perils of hundreds of millions of human lives, and future changemakers, will endure if we do not take actionable steps towards some tangible hope for the future."

—**Isabel Lu, Cornell University BS 2020 (Nutritional Sciences, Inequality**
Studies), University of North Carolina, Stillings (graduate studies, MPH, RD)

"Academic freedom is virtually sacred, and without it, students are denied the privilege of harnessing powerful information on nutrition that saves lives. In *The Future of Nutrition*, Dr. Campbell tells how institutional power, bias, and a reductionist system have resulted in a dangerously misinformed public on nutrition and health. It is vital we heed Campbell's call to continue to fight for the unobstructed freedom of science."

—**Jessie Stahl, Senior Policy and Program Coordinator,**
PlantPure Communities, Cornell University, BS 2017
(Nutritional Sciences), Duke University (Nursing Studies)

THE FUTURE

of

NUTRITION

An Insider's Look at the Science, Why We Keep Getting It Wrong, *and* How to Start Getting It Right

T. COLIN CAMPBELL, PhD

with NELSON DISLA

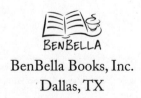

BenBella Books, Inc.
Dallas, TX

The Future of Nutrition copyright © 2020 by T. Colin Campbell

BenBella Books, Inc.
10440 N. Central Expressway
Suite 800
Dallas, TX 75231
www.benbellabooks.com
Send feedback to feedback@benbellabooks.com

BenBella is a federally registered trademark.

Printed in the United States of America
10 9 8 7 6 5 4 3 2 1

Library of Congress Cataloging-in-Publication Data:
Names: Campbell, T. Colin, 1934- author. | Disla, Nelson, editor.
Title: The future of nutrition : an insider's look at the science, why we keep getting it wrong, and how to start getting it right / T. Colin Campbell ; [edited by] Nelson Disla.
Description: Dallas, TX : BenBella Books, Inc., [2020] | Includes bibliographical references and index. | Summary: "Colin Campbell, author of The China Study (3M sold across all formats and editions) and New York Times bestseller Whole, returns with The Future of Nutrition, a book examining the shortcomings and confusion within the nutrition industry and outlining steps to improve"— Provided by publisher.
Identifiers: LCCN 2020028143 (print) | LCCN 2020028144 (ebook) | ISBN 9781950665709 (hardback) | ISBN 9781950665730 (ebook)
Subjects: LCSH: Nutrition. | Diet.
Classification: LCC RA784 .C23522 2020 (print) | LCC RA784 (ebook) | DDC 613.2—dc23
LC record available at https://lccn.loc.gov/2020028143
LC ebook record available at https://lccn.loc.gov/2020028144

Editing by Leah Wilson
Copyediting by James Fraleigh
Proofreading by Lisa Story and Sarah Vostok
Indexing by WordCo Indexing Services
Text design and composition by Aaron Edmiston

Cover design by Faceout Studio, Spencer Fuller
Cover photo © Shutterstock / Paladin12 (paper); Morphart Creation (kohlrabi); Little Apple (yam and mushrooms)
Printed by Lake Book Manufacturing

Distributed to the trade by Two Rivers Distribution, an Ingram brand
www.tworiversdistribution.com

To my initial personal acquaintances in the profession (about 1990–91), who were walking the talk with people and making meaningful my message from the research community (alphabetically): Antonia Demas, Hans Diehl, Caldwell Esselstyn, Alan Goldhamer, Doug Lisle, John McDougall, Dean Ornish, and Pam Popper.

And as always, to my immediate family: Karen; our five children Nelson, LeAnne, Keith, Dan, and Tom, and their spouses, Kim, Eva, Lisa, and Erin; and our eleven grandchildren, Whitney, Colin, Steven, Nelson, Laura, Kathryn, Mckenzie, Alistair, Skye, William, and Mira.

CONTENTS

PREFACE AND ACKNOWLEDGMENTS

Before I can share what I've learned about the science of nutrition, its past, and hopefully its future, there are so many people that I must acknowledge. Without these people, going all the way back to my youth, both my career and this book would have been impossible.

For context, it's important to emphasize that throughout my career in experimental research, I often encountered results that not only surprised me but also challenged many beliefs dear to both the public and my peers. Deciding to confront those beliefs was not always easy, even when the evidence was worth pursuing. For one thing, I did not want to jeopardize my financial support, which required professional peer approval. Neither did I want to be considered a fool. But despite those (and other) obstacles, some of the findings simply could not be ignored, for they had profound implications for our society's future.

It is here that I must first acknowledge the rock-solid support of my parents, who worked tremendously hard to raise me and my younger siblings while running a family dairy farm 365 days a year—cows don't take holidays! My mom kept a top-grade garden that provided most of our food year-round, and had me work in it when I was not in the barn or the fields working with my dad and brothers.

Dad, an immigrant from Northern Ireland, arrived at Ellis Island when he was only seven years old. He had a couple years of schooling, then worked very hard for the rest of his life. Because of his lack of formal schooling, he was exceptionally committed to the importance of education for his children. He wanted us to receive the education that he did not. He therefore did not want me to attend the local, rural high school, from which some students did not graduate and very few went to college. But the nearest really good tuition-free public high school was a little over fifty miles away, in Washington, DC. So, for five years, I drove our family car just over a hundred miles per day to attend that school. This allowed me to get a high-quality education at almost no expense (my uncle, whose small construction company lay along my route, paid for gas). Still, it was not easy to balance school and work on the farm. Because work usually awaited me after school each day, I had virtually no time to do homework, except for a study period during the school day.

After graduating high school, I passed through undergraduate school (pre-veterinary, Penn State), one year of veterinary school (University of Georgia), then graduate school (Cornell, master's and doctoral degrees in nutritional biochemistry). Several times along the way, I received generous, unsolicited offers of support by mentors and others. Many people, mostly professors and administrators, did generous favors for me, often uninvited and sometimes hardly knowing me. Without their collective generosity and goodwill, I might not have been the first on either side of my family to go to college.

How, then, did I come to pursue a professional career in nutrition and health that challenged such cherished beliefs concerning the food we eat, especially when those beliefs were such important parts of my upbringing? Did I not respect the discipline that gave me a professional career, and the people who helped me get there? Did I not respect the customs of my family, or the hardworking people in the farm community of my youth?

The research findings that drove my career were often culturally and economically challenging and disruptive. But they were also tied up in the personal story I have just described. Findings that questioned the health value of animal protein, as first (and repeatedly) indicated by experimental results showing that cow's-milk protein would be the most relevant chemical carcinogen ever, if it were officially tested, are culturally and economically challenging. But they were also personally challenging. Findings suggesting that nutrition plays a far greater role in cancer development than genetics were culturally and economically challenging. But they also challenged what I had been taught by people to whom I am still indebted. These findings challenged the entire status quo, the very one that had nurtured my career. There are many other examples—findings that undermined the pharmaceutical industry, or that showed experimental disease progression is reversible (i.e., treated) simply by removing its nutritional stimulus, or that the third- or fourth-leading (*but unlisted*) cause of death in America is the use of prescription drugs, or that optimal nutrition advances human health more than any combination of drugs, or that nutrition can both prevent *and* treat a wide range of illness and disease, with the benefits often appearing within days to weeks.

Thankfully, I felt I had no choice but to interpret our research findings to the best of my ability, no matter how provocative and challenging they were. When I think about that challenge, I think once more about my parents, especially my dad, who made sure I fully appreciated the combined power of work ethic and honesty. He reminded me more than once that I should "tell the truth, the whole truth, and nothing but the truth," and that reminder served me as armor more than once.

I believe that most people in science can relate to the spirit with which I pursued these research findings. That's why, for the most part, I've immensely enjoyed the scientific research community. Most of these scientists do not seek personal wealth. They are driven by curiosity, knowing that science, at its best, seeks truths in a way that leads to lively conversation. These experiences are very personal and social. Although I have experienced and treasured such exchanges, I also know that this is often not the public image of science, and for good reasons: scientists, unfortunately, are too often not at liberty to express their inner selves as a result of institutional expectations and boundaries. This is understandable within for-profit institutions, when scientists are contractually obliged and willing to stay within certain boundaries. But academic institutions are another thing altogether. They are endowed with *a public responsibility of seeking truths wherever they lead us*, whether in the research laboratory, the lecture hall, or policy boardrooms. Scientists are bound by a trust between academic institutions and the public to seek those truths, and when that trust is broken, all of society pays the price.

Sadly, there has been a serious drift away from these ideals in recent decades. The granting of academic tenure, and the freedom of speech and thought that it protects, has declined to such an extent that many of today's scientists in academia—especially in disciplines related to human health—are vulnerable. As of 2017, only 17 percent of US faculty were in tenured positions, and the proportion of non-tenured (adjunct) positions had quadrupled since 1975.[1] Most new faculty now have time-dependent terms of employment, which means that they may not be reappointed at the end of their term if they veer too far from the institutional "party line." Because they remain untenured, such faculty must be careful to not question their institutions' interests. To make matters even worse, most of those institutions are becoming increasingly tethered to external funding sources.

Though I discuss this threat at greater length later in this book, these acknowledgments would be incomplete without at least some mention of academic freedom. I was most fortunate to earn tenure exactly fifty years ago, in 1970. Without that privilege, this book and its predecessors would have never been written. I place it alongside parental guidance as another critical factor in my career.

But two-legged stools are not stable. The third leg is my wife of fifty-eight years, Karen. Though not trained in science, she had a more precious gift. She expressed it to me after we first met, simply stating that she did not tell lies. And such it has been. It was she, more than anyone else, who pressed me in 2002 to write my first book, *The China Study* (co-authored with our son, Tom, now a family physician). She and I are a team. She took up where my dad left off. With Karen by my side, I could never have failed to tell *the whole truth*, even if I were so inclined.

I muse on these matters of truth telling not because they are unique to me, but because they reflect some of the reasons why I followed the path I did in my research and academic career. That path was sometimes a delight, but also sometimes tortuous and bothersome. *The China Study* (2005, 2016) was written to share with the public some of the most provocative research that I could not ignore. *Whole* (2013) was written to explain the underlying philosophy and evidence that supported that research.

Here, I hope to answer another question: why does nutrition *still* struggle so much to be heard? I am not speaking only of recent struggles that I have faced personally, but of patterns that go back *centuries*. For me, though I didn't know it at the time, work on this book began in 1985 when I was on sabbatical at Oxford University, working with my colleagues Sir Richard Peto and Jill Boreham. I spent considerable time in Oxford and London libraries trying to understand why nutrition was so difficult to comprehend—for my colleagues in research, for colleagues in the food and health policy development arena, and for the public. I am therefore grateful to my colleagues for allowing me the time to do that research. The document I completed during that year, which summarized my findings on the respective histories of cancer and nutrition, was the initial basis for this book. A blurred copy of the document was faxed from Oxford (the first fax I ever saw), and I saved it for many years until it was retyped by Director of Digital Marketing Sarah Dwyer, allowing me to finally tell this story and explain how it relates to what I've learned over six-plus decades of research.

This brings me to the dozens of graduate students, undergraduate honors students, and postdoctoral students who studied and worked under my mentorship—without those experiences, both personal and professional, I would not be where I am. Senior technicians Marty Root, PhD, and Linda Youngman, PhD, who spent about fifteen years each running my laboratory, and Banoo Parpia, PhD, chief administrator of our research program in China, also deserve great credit. They made this and my earlier books possible. I am also indebted to my colleagues at large, including more than two dozen who worked in my laboratory, among them many visiting professors and senior scientists from China. From this group, I owe a special debt of gratitude to Chen Junshi, MD, PhD, who was the first Chinese senior scientist to visit the US, and who spent a year as a visiting professor in my laboratory before later serving as the co-director on the China project with me and two other colleagues, the aforementioned Sir Richard Peto of Oxford University and Dr. Li Junyao of China. Our partnership spanned more than twenty-five very active years. Sir Richard Peto was, and continues to be according to many, the world's leading biostatistician and epidemiologist. He and Dr. Jill Boreham at Oxford were primarily responsible for organizing, collating, and displaying the original data in an 896-page monograph, jointly published by Oxford University Press, Cornell University Press, and People's Publishing House of China.

Perhaps oddly, but seriously, I acknowledge those few individuals who represent powerful institutions in our society and who position themselves for private gain at the expense of public welfare. These individuals within universities acquire personal funding from corporate consultancies and outsized honoraria, sometimes also getting institutional funding to conduct focused research projects for the benefit of those same corporations. I acknowledge these individuals because they illustrate the danger of powerful institutions exerting control over academic research and government policy, mostly beyond public view. In my experience, such individuals illustrate an existential immorality that must be excised. We have extremely important things to do without having to suffer costly distractions and, at times, the threat of professional annihilation over such a fundamental thing as sharing the truth with others.

I am also grateful to the nonprofit organizations that have put science-based, whole food, plant-based nutrition at the center of their own operations, including the Center for Nutrition Studies (CNS), under the direction of Jenny Miller, Jason Warfe and staff, and now having as president my daughter LeAnne Campbell (PhD, Education and Curriculum Development)*; Plant Pure Communities, founded by my son Nelson, underwritten by CNS, and directed by Jody Kass†; and the CNS-partially underwritten research program at the University of Rochester Medical Center, run by my son Tom (MD) and his wife, Erin.‡

I must acknowledge family—twenty-two children, spouses, and grandchildren in my immediate family—who have not only put up with me and the time I spend on the computer, but who have also wholeheartedly adopted this whole food, plant-based lifestyle. Except for one who very occasionally may veer off course, they all eat this way. Eleven work professionally in various ways in this area. Their support has been priceless, in so many ways. Son Nelson's extensive review of the manuscript is very much appreciated. And grandson Nelson Disla, graduate of the University of North Carolina with highest honors, my "with" author—I can easily say that his writing skills are without peer, in my experience.

Lastly, I have the utmost professional and personal respect for the exceptional work of Leah Wilson, Alexa Stevenson, James Fraleigh, Alicia Kania, Monica Lowry, Jennifer Canzoneri, and everyone else at BenBella Books.

* www.nutritionstudies.org/courses/plant-based-nutrition
† www.plantpurecommunities.org
‡ Tom: www.urmc.rochester.edu/people/27426401-thomas-campbell; Erin: www.urmc.rochester.edu/people/22553782-erin-campbell

FOREWORD

Growing up during World War II on a large Montana dairy farm, I never doubted the value and quality of the food we were producing. I was sure the meat and milk from our farm were the keys to a healthy future. And when it came time to decide my future occupation, that upbringing was ingrained in my decision. Even though farming was not very profitable, I believed that our growing world population would make it so.

After deciding to be a food producer, my next step toward mastering agriculture was to get a college degree. So I attended Montana State University and obtained a BS degree in Agriculture Production. I was now prepared to take the food production world by storm.

Yet I soon became aware of a problem: millions of producers were selling to only a handful of buyers. My farm would have to get bigger or get out. So I got bigger: I eventually controlled thousands of acres of crops and owned thousands of cattle. My college lessons dictated my production processes: chemicals to control the weeds, factory feedlot to fatten slaughter cattle, and big equipment to grow and harvest grain. I did begin to notice that my soil quality was declining, and that our animals had become numbers instead of valued companions. But I was too busy to think much about these issues. If they were important, I thought, we'd have studied them at the university. Plus my personal life had become busy, too: I was married and had five children.

Then, everything changed. I lost feeling from the waist down and was diagnosed with a spinal tumor. Before my surgery to address the growth, the doctor told me that if the tumor was inside the spinal column, my odds of walking after the operation were about one in a million. This got my attention. The night before the operation, many things crossed my mind, including the worsening condition of the soil and my relationship with our animals. I resolved that no matter the outcome of the procedure, I would attempt to rectify these issues.

It turned out that the tumor *was* inside the spinal cord, but against all the odds I was able to walk out of the hospital. I considered it my miracle. Through it all, and during my lengthy recovery, I did not forget about the soil or the animals.

After the surgery, physical labor was beyond my ability. I found reading to be a great way to pass the long days. It was at that time when I first became aware of Dr. T. Colin Campbell, a researcher at Cornell University. But at that phase of my life, his work was a bridge too far for me.

During my recovery, I became convinced that my farming methods were causing significant environmental damage. I decided to become an organic farmer. When I shared this plan with my banker, however, he laughed and said the bank would not lend me any money unless it was cycled through local chemical dealers. Unable to change my farming methods, and burdened with debt, I had two choices: continue with conventional agriculture, or liquidate my operation. I chose the latter.

After a failed congressional campaign against a multi-term incumbent, I accepted a lobbying job with a small family-farm organization in Washington, DC. For a small-town boy from rural Montana, working in the halls of government was a real eye opener. Seeing the doings of Congress up close was very different from reading about them in a civics book.

While in Washington, I continued to eat much the same way as I had on the farm. But I was getting much less physical activity, and I was becoming as fat a market-ready hog. I knew I had to make a significant change or else I was a heart attack waiting to happen.

I recalled Dr. Campbell's work, and decided to change my eating without telling anyone. I became a plant eater while working for meat and dairy producers. Over time, I lost in excess of 100 pounds.

At about the same time, a new problem called mad cow disease was rearing its ugly head in England. The symptoms were similar to issues I had seen in cattle in confined feeding on my farm, and the cause was thought to be feeding animal waste to live cattle, a common practice in most US confined-feeding operations. Not only was this a big problem for animal agriculture, it was now thought that humans who ate infected meat could develop the disease. This issue had the potential to upend the multibillion-dollar animal feeding industry, and no amount of money was too much for the cattle industry to spend in protecting business as usual.

The foundation of science is truth, but the American diet is built on so many falsehoods that it is almost impossible to tell truth from mistruth. Corporate agriculture in no way wants to clarify this situation, or for American consumers to discover that what they believe to be true is really false. Their tried and proven strategy was to disrupt science and rely on herd mentality. Again, and again, we are told to go with the herd.

I was working for the Beyond Beef campaign when I met Dr. Campbell in my office for the first time. Both of us being farm boys, we established an instant rapport that continues to this day.

Soon after this meeting, Oprah Winfrey decided to do a show about mad cow disease. As one of the few addressing the public about this issue, I was invited to appear. With millions of viewers set to tune in, the cattle industry panicked. They were represented by a lobbyist I had worked with in Congress and knew very well, but he represented the industry poorly on the show. Oprah ultimately stated on the program that she would never again eat a burger. What a disaster for cattlemen! The industry was put into total disarray.

When the cattlemen recovered, some of them decided that one way to discourage media coverage of mad cow disease was to sue Oprah and me for millions of dollars. This legal experience lasted for years, but we won every time. The base of our defense was the work of Dr. Campbell and the China Study. Because the cattlemen could not find any flaw in the research linking animal protein and cancer, they were unable to base their suit on the facts. We prevailed in the eyes of the jury not just because of the right of free speech, but also because our statements were grounded in science and truth.

This same drive to document how the food, medical, and pharmaceutical industries, in conjunction with vested government interests, have worked to discredit the benefits of a plant-based diet can be found throughout Dr. Campbell's new book, *The Future of Nutrition*. While reading it, all I could think of was how much easier my transition away from animal-based foods would have been if this book had been available when I was becoming a plant eater. It's a pleasure to read truth from a truly gifted scientist.

I owe Dr. T. Colin Campbell a debt I will never be able to pay. In my view, he should receive the Nobel Peace Prize.

—Howard F. Lyman
Author, *Mad Cowboy*

INTRODUCTION

There are few things more provocative than the food we choose to eat, both in terms of its effect on health and people's sensitivity surrounding those choices. Any suggestion of dietary change is rife with potential agitation. This has been the case for at least four decades, and I have had the unusual "privilege" of witnessing and experiencing that agitation up close many times since my professional career began some sixty years ago. My experience includes thirteen years at MIT and Virginia Tech; one year each at Oxford University and the headquarters of the Federation of American Societies for Experimental Biology and Medicine (FASEB) in the Washington, DC, area, where I was US Congressional liaison representative for the Federation; and forty-five years at my alma mater, Cornell. From all of that experience, one episode in particular stands out for its ability to illustrate the sensitivity and controversy surrounding nutrition.

In 1980, I was invited by the US National Academy of Sciences (NAS) to join a thirteen-member expert panel tasked with studying the relationship of diet and nutrition with cancer. Three years earlier, a US Senate committee chaired by Senator George McGovern had released a landmark report on diet and heart disease. Its dietary goals were ultimately modest, encouraging things like lower dietary fat intake and greater consumption of fruits and vegetables.[1] Nevertheless, the report triggered hostile reactions from the immensely powerful and wealthy food industry. Senator McGovern told me some years later that this report was the proudest achievement in his public life, but it wasn't won easily. Six of his Senate colleagues lost their 1980 reelection efforts as a result of their support for the report's findings, he said. They were from farm states, where agribusiness exerts serious influence on the political process.

Naturally, the public wanted to know whether diet might have a similar effect on other common diseases, especially cancer. The question was reasonable enough: Might the dietary recommendations best suited for controlling heart disease also be consistent with controlling cancer? The authority on this question should have been Dr. Arthur Upton, director of the US National Cancer Institute (NCI)—a subdivision of the US National Institutes of Health (NIH)—who was invited to testify before the Senate.* Unfortunately, Dr. Upton was unable to answer the question to anyone's satisfaction, and instead revealed NCI's negligent attitude toward nutrition research. When asked how much of his budget was devoted to nutrition, Upton replied, "2–3 percent." The Senate responded in early 1980 by appropriating $1 million to the NCI for a review of the literature on nutrition and cancer. The NCI in turn contracted with the NAS to conduct the study. This was organized by Dr. Sushma Palmer of the NAS and Dr. Peter Greenwald, director of the new Division of Cancer Prevention at NCI, both of whom expressed interest in research on the nutrition–cancer connection.

Political considerations were immediately intense and ugly, even just in deciding which group should write the report, highlighting once again how controversial such a report could be. Within the NAS (situated just down the street from the Capitol and embedded amid large marble structures of national power both descript and nondescript), the Food and Nutrition Board (FNB) immediately jockeyed for control. This is the same group that has been tasked every five years since the early 1940s with estimating and publishing recommended daily allowances (RDAs) for individual nutrients. As far as they were concerned, preparation of the nutrition and cancer report was both their institution's right and responsibility. They also knew how incendiary a report on this topic could be. But the decision wasn't theirs to make. Concerned about several of the FNB members' food industry

---

* Dr. Upton sent his proposed testimony to me and our Division of Nutritional Sciences director at Cornell for our comments prior to his presentation.

associations, Dr. Phil Handler, the president of the NAS at that time, opted for a new, outside committee of experts—that thirteen-member panel to which I was invited.

As you can imagine, the FNB wasn't thrilled by this decision. In what I came to understand as an attempt to usurp our report and preemptively undermine whatever conclusions we might make, they published their own twenty-four-page report, titled "Toward Healthful Diets,"[2] in 1980, just as we began our work. Here is a brief excerpt:

> *In the case of diseases with multiple and poorly understood etiology, such as cancer and cardiovascular disease, the assumption that dietary change will be effective as a preventive measure is controversial. These diseases are not primarily nutritional, although they have nutritional determinants that vary in importance from individual to individual . . .*
>
> *Those experts who . . . seek to change the national diet in the hope of preventing these degenerative diseases assume that the risk of change is minimal and rely heavily on epidemiologic evidence for support of their belief in the probability of benefit. Neither the degree of risk nor the extent of benefit can be assumed in the absence of suitable evidence . . .*
>
> *The Board expresses its concerns over excessive hopes and fears in many current attitudes toward food and nutrition. Sound nutrition is not a panacea. Good food that provides appropriate proportions of nutrients should not be regarded as a poison, a medicine, or a talisman. It should be eaten and enjoyed.*

It may not be obvious to those unfamiliar with nutrition policy, but this report is pregnant with all manner of nuance and commentary intended to protect the status quo—the status quo that McGovern's report, and ours, threatened to upend. It first cleverly admits a few widely held understandings (e.g., disease causation is poorly understood, dietary change will be controversial, individual responses will vary, excessive hopes and fears arising from dietary change are concerning) that could serve as a means to shut down any nutritional recommendations. The report then posits that the adults in the room are its authors, that they are more reasonable and protective of the public than anyone else could possibly be, and that they know best—thereby shutting down any outside attempts at proposals for public benefit that might challenge corporate interests.

In one sense, the authors of this passage were absolutely correct: "that dietary change will be effective as a preventive measure *is* controversial" (emphasis added). But to imply that the controversy generated by dietary recommendations in any way undermines those recommendations' truthfulness is a clearly faulty premise. No matter how controversial any evidence may be, the controversy itself is never enough to rule that evidence out. Moreover, "controversy" does not necessarily mean that contradicting evidence exists. The notion that smoking causes cancer was once viewed as extremely controversial, not because of an impressive body of evidence proving the healthfulness of tar and nicotine, but because it challenged prevailing norms. The notion that huge industries like the pharmaceutical and food industries "make a killing" by selling their products to a population that only becomes more ill as a result is controversial—and it should be! Evidence that disputes the status quo will *always* be controversial, whether it is true or not, because that's the very definition of controversy: disagreement over conventional understanding. Interestingly enough, the same definition could apply to all of science—if a theory cannot be scientifically disputed, refuted, or falsified, it is often viewed as pseudoscience. In other words, controversy is the sound that science makes. To downplay scientific evidence because it is controversial is to downplay scientific evidence for the very same, fundamental reason that science is celebrated.

The "outsiders" panel on which I sat worked on our report for three years and included six three-day conferences and considerable staff input. The report had two parts: a 478-page summary of the available scientific evidence,[3] then 74 pages of recommendations on research needs.[4] Once published in 1982, it quickly became the most sought-after report in the history of the NAS. This was both a blessing and a curse. On the one hand, the level of interest our report generated verified the public's interest in this message and the importance of the topic. On the other, the attention that followed was not without consequences. Like the McGovern report that preceded it, our work—though modest, in my opinion—enraged authorities in the food industry, their consultants, and their apologists in academic science communities. One prominent voice, Professor Tom Jukes of the University of

California, even lamented the moment as "the day that food was declared a poison."[5]

Within two weeks, the industry-controlled* Council for Agricultural Science and Technology (CAST) retaliated with a summary[6] of their own, which included the critical views of forty-five scientists (forty-two university faculty for added authority). Most were beholden to the agriculture industry. Some were prominent members of the aforementioned FNB, which had been excluded from writing the nutrition–cancer report. For good measure, copies of the critique were placed on the desks of each and every one of the 535 legislators of the US Senate and House of Representatives. Congress was thus served skepticism on a golden platter by a seemingly legitimate group of scientific authorities—and through them, so too was the public.

Additionally, I learned that the American Institute of Nutrition (AIN, now the American Society for Nutrition), a society of professional nutrition researchers of which I was a member in good standing, was angered by our committee's report. I became especially aware of this after being featured in a then relatively new consumer magazine, *People*; appearing on PBS's *McNeill-Lehrer NewsHour*; and giving expert testimony before House and Senate committees. This increasing visibility made me an easy and obvious target among my professional nutrition science community, and the AIN quickly set about making an example of me. First, my nomination by the executive council and election as the AIN president was aborted.† Next, the society revoked my nomination for its most prestigious award. Last and most significantly, the AIN's two most influential members filed a petition to expel me from the society. Although a formal hearing in Washington, DC, eventually and unanimously cleared me of any wrongdoing, it was clear that I had broken a few too many unspoken rules. Expulsion from the AIN would have been devastating to my reputation given that it was the only

---

* Established in 1972, CAST is a nonprofit 501(c)(3) organization that, according to its mission statement, "assembles, interprets, and communicates credible, balanced, science-based information to policy makers, the media, the private sector, and the public." Among its many sustaining members, you probably recognize several stalwarts of credibility and science-based information, including Bayer CropScience, the Coca-Cola Company, Land O'Lakes, Tyson Foods, and the preposterously named Merck Animal Health.

† According to an AIN staff member who was privy to the vote count.

professional organization of its kind, requiring a doctorate in nutrition and the publication of at least five peer-reviewed papers. In fact, I had the strange honor of being the target of the first expulsion effort in the society's history.

Ultimately, the AIN's attempts to besmirch me, nasty though they were, amounted to little more than petulance. As angry and shocked as I was at the time, I'm thankful for them now. I would not be where I am today without such episodes, and I wouldn't trade my place for anything. The reason I share them now is to illustrate just how sensitive our institutions are and how vengeful they can become when the conventional knowledge they espouse, and their authority to do so, are challenged.

Perhaps the most surprising aspect of this fracas was that the dietary goals outlined in our NAS report were quite moderate. As in the McGovern report before us, we recommended decreased dietary fat intake and increased consumption of fruits, vegetables, and whole grains. Although I insisted that the report include a chapter on the association between protein and cancer—a major focus in my work and in this book—and prepared the main draft for that chapter, this was meant primarily to encourage future research, and the report made no recommendations about eliminating meat products from the diet.[3] But even the inclusion of this section on protein was too much for most of the other committee members. I was later told by a colleague on the AIN Council, who was privy to the aborted presidential election and expulsion attempt, that I had "fundamentally betrayed" the interests of the nutrition research community. I had done this by publishing nutrition research that was not within the realm of "acceptable" knowledge, even though the research was twice vetted by professional peer review, once to acquire research funding and once to publish it in professional journals.

To build on the earlier point, then, evidence that threatens the status quo *in nutrition research* will always be controversial, whether it is true or not. The evidence in favor of reducing the intake of dietary fat was controversial then, and remains so now. Even without dietary recommendations on the subject, the mere inclusion of a chapter about protein and cancer was extremely controversial.

In the time since, I have seen many examples of how the scientific community selectively prohibits certain "controversial" subjects (when they threaten the status quo) from discussion. Even before the 1982 report, I witnessed and experienced much the same timidity of thought and stagnation in the sciences of cancer and nutrition. In virtually every arena of science, including laboratory settings, classrooms, health policy boardrooms, and public lecture halls, I witnessed the same patterns. More often than I care to remember, I felt pressured to quit asking controversial questions and "return to the flock" (something I have discussed to some degree in previous books, especially *The China Study* and *Whole*).

The question this book will be asking is: *Why?* Why was it that the subject of animal protein in particular came to be forbidden from the study and discourse of nutrition? Why was it that nutrition came to be forbidden from the study and discourse of cancer? Why are these such incendiary issues in the first place?

HARNESSING THE CONTROVERSY OF THE WHOLE FOOD, PLANT-BASED DIET

The research I presented in *The China Study* and expanded in *Whole*, both from my career and from the careers of others, supports the adoption of a whole food, plant-based (WFPB) diet for the promotion of health and the prevention and treatment of disease. My research has been a deep source of controversy, which I believe offers a unique case study of the many challenges and opportunities facing science and our society as a whole. But let's take a moment first to review what I mean when I refer to a WFPB diet.

At its simplest and most accessible, the WFPB diet can be described in a dozen words, distilled into two recommendations:

1. Consume a variety of whole plant-based foods.
2. Avoid consumption of animal-based foods.

A WFPB diet is not the same thing as a vegan diet, which is defined by what it eliminates: animal foods. A WFPB diet is defined also by what it emphasizes: a variety of whole plant foods. By *whole*, I mean all a food's nutrients are consumed together, regardless of whether the foods are diced, sliced, cooked, or blended. I also mean that added oils and refined carbohydrates such as table sugar should be used sparingly if at all. So-called convenience foods like potato chips are not whole. High in refined ingredients, they undermine health in every respect: they are calorically replete, nutrient deficient, and absolutely *inconvenient* in the long term. (Or can you imagine a scenario in which sudden coronary death is convenient?)*

I offer these dietary recommendations for optimal health on the basis of a wide range of evidence. This evidence includes:

- experimental laboratory-animal studies that observed a strong and mostly causal association between modestly high consumption of animal protein (anything in excess of about 10 percent of calories) and cancer—an effect that was not observed in the consumption of plant protein;
- experimental laboratory-animal studies that found at least ten mechanisms by which this animal protein effect was working, both in the early initiation phase and later promotion phase of cancer (adding what researchers call "biological plausibility," and suggesting that the cancer growth was not being caused by something else);
- a wide range of international correlation studies that show a linear correlation of animal protein with multiple cancers, cardiovascular disease, and other chronic diseases;
- human intervention studies that have demonstrated the reversal of heart disease by a diet absent of animal protein and composed of whole plant-based foods;
- and other corroborating evidence.

No other diet has ever been shown to not only prevent but also reverse heart disease, and there exist no large-scale, international correlation studies

---

* Though it will be covered in greater depth later, the subject of weight control often arises in discussions of a WFPB diet. It has been widely presumed that the WFPB dietary regimen requires no calorie counting, and in most cases I agree that this is not necessary. However, for those who are unable to lose body weight and sustain its loss, it should be noted that consuming excess calories, usually in the form of calorie-dense foods (e.g., nuts or avocados), or failing to get enough exercise, are also important considerations.

that show the opposite effect (increased animal protein consumption associated with decreased heart disease, cancer, etc.).

Moreover, there are virtually no nutrients contained in animal foods that are not better provided by plant foods. The adjoining chart shows the relative amounts of nutrients found in intact plant and animal foods for five nutrient groups. The differences are huge, as are their relative effects on health. Antioxidants, complex carbohydrates, and vitamins, all unique to plants,* have been repeatedly shown to prevent and treat heart disease, cancer, and other chronic degenerative diseases when consumed in whole foods (not supplements). Additionally, plant foods easily provide the necessary intakes of fat and protein long recommended by authoritative institutions, rather than the excessive amounts provided by animal foods.†

Nutrient Compositions*

COMPONENT	PLANT	ANIMAL
Antioxidants	Only Made By Plants	Almost None
Complex Carbs	Only Made By Plants	None
Vitamins	Made By Plants	Almost None
Fat	~9–11%	~15–20%
Protein	~9–11%	~15–20%

*PROCESSED FOODS are varied, likely worse.

This compelling body of evidence in favor of a WFPB diet has already been surveyed and interpreted at much greater length in other books, including *The China Study*, so I will not cover it comprehensively here. My point is that I have been privileged to share this evidence for many years, through books (*The*

---

* Vitamin A (the animal-based retinol) is, by definition, not a vitamin because our bodies produce all the retinol we need when we consume the beta carotene produced by plants—beta carotene is the real vitamin A. Likewise, our bodies produce "vitamin D" given the right amount of sun exposure—deficiency is only a problem for those living closer to the poles.

† Certain plants (nuts and avocado, for example) are higher in fat, but their activities when ingested as a whole food are far more beneficial than when ingested as isolated oils and fats.

China Study, Whole, and *The Low-Carb Fraud*), documentary films (*Forks over Knives* and *PlantPure Nation*), and nearly a thousand public and professional lectures around the world since *The China Study* was published in 2005 (and many, many more before then). And what I have learned during this time, and especially since I began to share this information more publicly in 2005, is that the WFPB diet is fascinatingly controversial among certain groups.

I believe there are three primary reasons for this controversy:

1. The WFPB diet and its supporting research findings challenge the conventional understanding of **disease**, both its causes and treatments. This is especially true of cancer, long regarded as a genetic disease triggered by environmental carcinogens, not poor nutrition. Likewise, the treatments for cancer considered best practice have traditionally been invasive, targeted protocols— surgery, radiation, and chemotherapy—versus nutritional treatment (which admittedly needs additional discriminating research). The WFPB diet and its supporting evidence could seriously undermine these long-held beliefs and practices.

2. The WFPB diet and its supporting research findings challenge the conventional understanding of **nutrition** itself, especially orthodox attitudes toward animal protein, which has long been regarded as the most influential nutrient and has played a determining role in our dietary preferences.

3. Perhaps most fundamentally, the WFPB diet and its supporting research findings challenge the conventional understanding of what reliable **science** and scientific evidence look like. Modern science is increasingly specialized, reductionist, and bent toward the production of technological solutions. In "nutrition science," this means the production of pharmaceutical solutions and nutrient supplements. The WFPB diet is controversial because it disputes this prevailing norm and demands a more *wholistic* view of evidence.

When we dissect these points of controversy, a bigger picture emerges about how and why our institutions codify what kinds of science—what hypotheses, research proposals, and data interpretations—are (and are not) accepted for funding, publication, and policy development. This, in turn, impacts both the way in which we (mis)use past science and the possibilities for future science. In short, by investigating the three points of controversy above, we can learn a great deal about the entanglement of science and institutions—from academic institutions such as Cornell University, to professional institutions such as the AIN, to public policy agencies and advisories such as the Dietary Guidelines Advisory Committee.

I am excited to elaborate on this controversy and institutional dysfunction because it transcends the subjects of the WFPB diet, nutrition, and even science in general. In nutrition, it has led to mass confusion about the most scientifically justified approach to eating, and even about how nutrition operates, with devastating consequences for our society's health. But it also has a tremendous impact on other fields and raises questions of great importance for politics and ethics. The institutional dysfunction that I am describing has led not only to excessive health care costs and imposing environmental problems, but also to mass public and professional confusion, disillusionment, and disengagement.

A ROADMAP

This book is organized around the three areas of controversy listed above. We will look at each of them in turn, to bring into greater focus the challenges facing nutrition, science, and the health of all society. We will then conclude with a number of suggestions for how we might evolve and restore function to the institutions affecting science (funding, publication, education, etc.), thus changing the future of nutrition—empowering the public to better their health, the health of their communities, and the health of the planet.

My primary hope is not that everyone reading this book will eat the same diet that I eat (though I would obviously recommend it), for I think the themes and implications of this investigation are of an even greater, universal concern. The reason I devote this particular book to discussing the science of nutrition is not to pigeonhole these topics, but because it is the science to which I have been dedicated for more than six decades. Likewise, the reason

I discuss the controversy generated by the WFPB diet is not to alienate or convert anyone, but because I cannot possibly escape that controversy, and because it offers the most profound case study of institutional dysfunction that I could possibly imagine.

In that spirit, I am not interested here in debunking fad diets, advertising superfoods and quick fixes, or heaping onto the controversy that already exists. Rather, I want to embrace what controversy exists and admit it for inspection—not because controversial evidence is patently false, but because controversy is the inevitable result of challenges to the status quo. I would like to make sense of the origin and promotion of this controversy because of what is at stake. When it comes to human health, the status quo is an ugly thing: every day, human lives are impoverished, disabled, and ended by avoidable diseases. Is that a status quo worth preserving? And so, I return to the controversy to make sense of it, so that we might begin to make sense of ourselves.

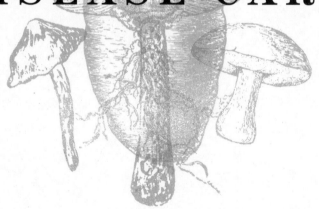

PART I

CHALLENGING
DISEASE CARE

CHAPTER ONE

DISEASE CARE TODAY

Nothing is more expensive than a missed opportunity.
—H. Jackson Brown Jr.

W e can no longer deny it—the health of our society is in critical condition and has been for quite some time. The culprit?
Preventable lifestyle-related diseases—including heart disease,
stroke, cancer, type II diabetes, obesity, kidney disease, rheumatoid arthritis,
and any other disease for which the patient's outcome is strongly associated
with lifestyle choices such as diet—and a fundamental misunderstanding in
our society about where these diseases come from.

Chances are that you, like the vast majority of the population, have had
firsthand experiences with one or more of these diseases. Perhaps you have
lost friends or family to heart disease, stroke, or cancer, or maybe battled these
or other diseases yourself. These are the villains of real-life horror stories, and
their cost to society, both in dollars spent and lives lost, cannot be overstated.

The lives prematurely lost to heart disease alone—647,000 every year—boggle the mind. That's more than the population of many American cities, including Baltimore, Memphis, Atlanta, Miami, Albuquerque, and Sacramento. Can you imagine losing the equivalent population of one of those cities, each and every year, for the foreseeable future? Imagine the public outcry if 647,000 Americans died every year in a needless war against an invented enemy. Worse yet, imagine if it were already happening and no one addressed it! *And that's* only *heart disease.* What about other preventable diseases? The Centers for Disease Control and Prevention (CDC) lists the top five causes of death in 2017[1] as heart disease (647,000), cancer (599,000), accidents (170,000), chronic lower respiratory disease (160,000), and stroke (146,000). But here's the kicker: these are not inevitable deaths. Estimates suggest that up to 90 percent of heart disease deaths,[2] 70 percent of cancer deaths,[3] and 50 percent of stroke deaths,[3] plus my estimate of 80 percent of medical error deaths (more surgeries and cancer treatments = more chances for mishaps), could be prevented by informed use of nutrition.

That these diseases could be prevented offers hope—and it should—but also condemns our current approaches. If so much suffering and its attendant costs could be prevented through better nutrition, then why have we not done so? Have we forgotten that these are more than just numbers, that these are lives lost prematurely and families left behind? Like you, I know this personally. In March 1969, my mother-in-law discovered blood in her stool and went to the hospital, where she was seen by a doctor before being promptly sent home with a laxative. With no money (or insurance), no knowledge of her problem, and no information on how she might have avoided the problem, she was the victim of a broken system. She did not tell her daughter—my wife—or get the opinion of another doctor. By the time we did know, nine months later when she returned to the hospital, it was too late. This time she received a proper diagnosis: advanced colon cancer. Barely older than fifty, she spent the following three months, the final three months of her life, in the hospital. In March 1970, a year after that first appointment, she passed.

Two years later, while I was working in the Philippines, my father passed prematurely as a result of cardiovascular disease. My mother and a family friend had to travel over country roads to bring him to the nearest hospital, about twenty minutes away, and he never made it. I was shocked. Here was a man who was not overweight, who spent many hours working outdoors on the farm, and who ate what was considered to be a healthy American diet—a model of the "good" behavior encouraged at the time—and yet he died anyway.

Little has changed in the decades since. If anything, disease has become an even more normal part of American life, as illustrated by the continued growth of the pharmaceutical industry. In 2017, the average American's out-of-pocket pharmaceutical costs (including for those covered by insurance) amounted to a shocking $1,162.[4] Fifty-five percent of Americans take prescription drugs—four per day, on average[5]—and many of these people, as well as many of the minority who do not regularly take prescription drugs, take dietary supplements, too. We are also one of only two countries in the world that permits direct-to-consumer TV advertising of drugs, instead of advertising only to qualified physicians.* By any measure, we are fixated on magic pills, certainly more than any other country in the world. This does not suggest health, but rather the normalcy of disease.

National Trends in Per Capita Phamaceutical Spending, 1980-2015

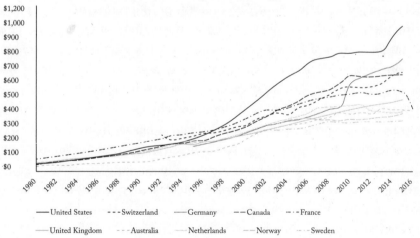

—— United States   - - - Switzerland   .... Germany   — — Canada   — · · France

—— United Kingdom   - - · Australia   ——— Netherlands   — — Norway   · · · · Sweden

---

* As of this writing, I was told by an interviewer in New Zealand, the other country where they allow direct-to-consumer advertising, that her country is in the process of changing their regulations.[6]

Along with our current approach to treatment, the economic costs of preventable disease are unsustainable. And they are rising: in 2020, health care costs occupy nearly 18 percent of our national budget, more than three times greater than in 1960 (5 percent), and total $3.5 trillion.[7] According to a PBS television program that reported on a comprehensive survey of health care,[8] the US pays two-and-a-half times more, per capita, for health care than thirty-five similarly affluent countries (members of the international Organisation for Economic Co-operation and Development).[9] This is not the result of higher infrastructure or labor costs, as some might expect. In fact, the US only has 2.4 physicians and 2.6 hospital beds per 1,000 people, both of which are less than the average among its OECD sister countries (3.1 physicians and 3.4 hospital beds per 1,000 people). Using these averages,[9] I calculate that the US spends a far greater proportion of its health care costs on pills than similar countries (approximately 3.3 times more). This estimate, which I call a "drug intensity index," reflects an unrivaled, historic emphasis on using drugs as the principal means of health care.

And how effective has this approach been? From my perspective, not effective at all. Although many commentators among the public and the media point to statistics on *life expectancy* as proof positive of our improved health, these statistics should be taken with a grain of salt. Life expectancy as a simple indicator of our health is limited. It's important to know not only *how long* we expect to live but also *how well*. Long life coupled with disabling, painful disease that exacts a heavy toll on family resources is not what most people want. All the same, changes in life expectancy do comprise an important part of our collective health history and deserve some attention. During the past two centuries, when most Western countries were transitioning from poverty to affluence, life expectancy greatly increased. This is because total *mortality* decreased, mostly due to a reduction in childhood infectious diseases.[10] Starting in 1840, life expectancy increased at a rate of three months per year, until the 1950s and '60s, at which point the rate of increase slowed to two months per year (once we had reduced mortality from infectious diseases, there was less potential for extending lifespan).

Our life expectancy continued to increase at a rate of two months per year, from seventy-one years in 1960 to more than seventy-eight years in

2014.[11] But in 2015, the rate of increase dropped by half, to only 1.2 months for that year. This sparked concern, though some thought it was a statistical fluke. Not so. For the next three years (2016–2018), average life expectancy actually *decreased*, from 78.8 years to 78.6 years—the longest sustained decline in expected lifespan since 1915–1918, when the decline was "partially attributed to the casualties of World War I and the devastating 1918 influenza pandemic."[12] A decline in life expectancy of 0.2 years may not seem very impressive, but it is nonetheless highly statistically significant. In a population of 300 million, 0.2 fewer years of life expectancy translates to six million people failing to live an extra ten years, or three million people failing to live an extra twenty years.*

The director of the CDC called this backslide in life expectancy "a wakeup call."[13] Many have linked it to increasing rates of drug overdoses and suicides, but I would argue that these deaths do not occur in a vacuum, and may also be partly linked to preventable lifestyle-related diseases. Chronic preventable disease is a chronic drain on our quality of life, and thus has a profound negative impact on psychological wellness, which feeds overdose and suicide. Some may counter that overdose and suicide are more closely related to economic hardship than health concerns, but again, these phenomena are closely entwined, as illustrated by the overwhelming cost of health care. Disease is expensive, especially chronic disease.

In a nationwide study published in the *American Journal of Medicine*, Harvard and Ohio University researchers found that 62.1 percent of all bankruptcies in 2007 could be attributed to medical expenses.[14] It gets worse. Three-quarters of those debtors had health insurance and most "were well educated, owned homes, and had middle-class occupations." In other words, the system is so broken that even well-off people end up with unmanageable debt. Where does that leave the less fortunate, who are disproportionately affected by lifestyle diseases? Compared to a study conducted in 2001—just six years prior—"the share of bankruptcies attributable to medical problems rose by 49.6 percent." These figures are scandalous, but not surprising when you consider the rising costs of standard treatment. It costs at least $20,000

---

* The derivation of this number was contributed by a friend, Damon Demas, PhD, a professional mathematician.

per year to treat heart disease with stents and statins, and the average cost of one round of chemotherapy ranges from $20,000 (office-managed) to $26,000 (hospital-managed).[15]

Still, life expectancy *did* improve up until 2015. Surely that's a sign of progress, right? Yes and no. Some may be surprised to know that our increasing life expectancy from the '60s until recently is not due to improved health as much as improved strategies for responding to disease events. More and more people suffering from cancer, stroke, obesity, and diabetes are able to live longer with their diseases than before. Improved survival rates have been especially significant for those who suffer heart attacks. Indeed, about 60 percent of our increase in total life expectancy since 1960 can be attributed to improved rapid response in heart disease alone.[16] Yet our overall health has not improved significantly during this time. Incidence rates (new cases of disease) have remained relatively stable for heart disease and stroke, declined slightly for cancers (mostly because of less smoking-related lung cancer), and increased for diabetes (associated with our increased rate of obesity). Improvement in personal living conditions (for example, improved access to programs in stress management, physical conditioning, and routine medical care) following diagnosis has resulted in a modest increase in years of life lived with disease, but not the eradication of disease.[10,17]

Putting all of these trends together, one might tentatively argue that we have improved our treatment of disease. By responding to crises more quickly and improving living conditions, we manage our morbidity better than before. But we have not addressed the underlying causes of these diseases, or given any attention to the possibility of developing more effective means of treating and even reversing disease other than with the use of pharmaceuticals. The result is many more people requiring care, which has increased the burden on our health care system. This phenomenon could be called a failure of success, and it may get far worse yet. Some may point out that rising drug costs, which for a long time outpaced total health care costs, have slowed down as of 2019, but, as a proportion of total health care costs, drug costs in the US are still much higher than in other OECD countries.[18] As long as we remain dependent on those drugs to maintain life, without examining the factors affecting disease prevalence, we will continue to suffer the financial and quality of life consequences. This "failure of success" is no true success at all; true success would combine an increased life expectancy with less disease. Still, the parade marches on.

Despite some improvement in the *management* of disease, the struggle to treat disease remains elusive. One of the main reasons for this continued struggle has already been introduced: our outsized dependence on drugs, which attack symptoms without addressing their lifestyle roots, and divert resources and attention away from other strategies. Moreover, these drugs are causing a health crisis of their own:

- According to a report by Donald Light of the Safra Center for Ethics at Harvard, "Few people know that prescription drugs have a 1 in 5 chance of serious reactions *after* they have been approved" (emphasis added), and approximately 2.74 million hospitalizations per year can be attributed to adverse drug effects, not even including cases of misprescription, overdose, and self-medication.[19]
- "About 81 million adverse reactions are experienced by the 170 million Americans taking drugs."[19]
- According to a report by Public Citizen's Health Research Group, "Every day more than 4,000 patients have adverse drug reactions so serious that they need to be admitted to American hospitals."[20]
- In 2014, according to WebMD's citation of *Consumer Reports*,[5] nearly 1.3 million people "sought emergency room treatment for adverse effects of prescription drugs and about 124,000 people died."
- Prescription drug use is the fourth leading cause of death in the US, an estimate similar to a 1998 estimate by Starfield.[21] According to a 2018 US Food and Drug Administration report, annual US deaths from adverse effects of prescription drugs are estimated to be 106,000.[22]

The counterargument to these startling figures is that we need to balance the rate of adverse drug-related incidents against the number of individuals who benefit from drug use (i.e., efficacy) if we are going to properly assess the usefulness of drugs. As one report states, "if we suppose that all [170 million estimated drug users in 2014] benefit [from drug use], then the 2.7 million severe reactions is only about 1.5%."[19] However, this is a very low estimate of adverse reactions and it supposes that *all* users are benefiting from their drugs (an outrageously optimistic assumption). Nor does it consider adverse reactions that do not result in hospitalization, of which there are thirty times more.[19]

Of course, I don't mean to underplay the medical advances we have made over the last few decades, especially the rewards of faster response times. It's good to know that today my father would likely be able to get to the hospital much more quickly. Likewise, I'm impressed by the caretakers throughout our health care system. According to the Kaiser Family Foundation, there are over thirteen million such folks: neighbors, friends, professional specialists, and health care workers of all kinds.[23] I'm certain that virtually all of them are dedicated and compassionate servants of health. But overall, we're struggling. Our declining life expectancy leaves America ranked forty-fourth in the world,[24] an astonishing and disturbing rank considering that we have the highest per capita health care costs in the world, by an eye-popping margin. How do we reconcile our massive medical bills with such a low rank? Considering all of these trends and statistics simultaneously—very high drug use, declining life expectancy, and unusually low rank in life expectancy—it's hard to believe that we are on the right path.

And neither will this issue resolve itself. Virtually all reports advocating the use of pharmaceuticals are driven by the profit motive, and the profit has been undeniable. In 2017, global pharmaceutical revenue totaled $1.143 trillion, with a projected growth rate of 4.1 percent.[25] That's more than the revenues of national government budgets in *all but five* countries.[26] With such wealth comes tremendous power, and with that power, even greater influence on public and professional perceptions. In short, as long as the pharmaceutical industry continues to profit from our disease, crouched beneath the God of Fertile Markets, our questionable dependency on drugs will perpetuate itself, no matter how ineffective this approach has proven to be. Unless we do something about it, the health of our society will worsen still.

THE ROLE OF MALNUTRITION

The answer, then, isn't more or better drugs. It is understanding and addressing the primary culprit behind many of these diseases: malnutrition.

Malnutrition is a word I use advisedly. Although the word is usually reserved for descriptions of diets that are calorie deficient or missing certain essential nutrients, its literal meaning (faulty nutrition) also applies to dietary patterns of excess, which pose a much greater threat to most Americans.* This includes many Americans living in poverty. The poorest members of our society generally consume foods higher in simple sugars and excess oils, both of which contribute to obesity and higher risk for diabetes and cardiovascular disease, because these foods tend to be cheaper. Research going back many decades, including the landmark, decades-long Framingham Heart Study,[27] has linked heart disease with various risk factors, including high blood cholesterol and high blood pressure, that are symptoms of malnutrition. Furthermore, a combination of international[28] and migration studies[29-31] suggests that diet, as an environmental factor, plays not a minor role but in fact *the most significant* role in heart disease risk. Corroborating experimental research verified this more than sixty years ago: in a 1946–1958 study, Dr. Lester Morrison[32] split a group of heart attack survivors into two groups, one control and one experimental. In the experimental group, he instructed patients to reduce their consumption of fat and dietary cholesterol from 80–160 grams of fat and 200–1,800 milligrams of dietary cholesterol to 20–25 grams of fat and 50–70 milligrams of dietary cholesterol. After twelve years, every patient in the control group was dead, while 38 percent of the experimental group had survived. More recent research[2,33] suggests that this 38 percent survival rate can be elevated much further (upward of 90 percent), given a more complete dietary shift than the low-fat protocol designed by Morrison (in his study, for example, patients were still allowed to eat small amounts of lean meat). Nevertheless, the results could not have been clearer: *what we eat plays a significant role*

---

* Although I characterize Americans' dietary patterns as excessive, it is also true that certain deficiencies are common. Many Americans suffer from a lack of fiber and vitamins and minerals that are only found in plants.

in determining heart disease outcomes. Similar forms of evidence, including international correlation studies, migration studies, and experimental laboratory animal studies, have similarly linked diet with cancer, diabetes, obesity, kidney disease, and more.

By incorporating this research, and conservative estimates of the potential influence of malnutrition—which, as we saw earlier, suggests that massive numbers of deaths from heart disease,[2] cancer,[3] stroke,[3] and medical errors (assuming decreased need for drugs and other medical interventions that provide opportunity for such errors) could be prevented by good nutrition*— you can see the CDC's previously introduced list of the top causes of death transform.

Top Causes of Death in 2017	Adjusted for Malnutrition
Heart Disease: 647,000	Heart Disease: 65,000
Cancer: 599,000	Cancer: 180,000
Accidents: 170,000	Accidents: 170,000
Chronic Lower Respiratory: 160,000	Chronic Lower Respiratory: 160,000
Stroke: 146,000	Stroke: 73,000
Medical Errors: 250,000–440,000	Medical Errors: 50,000
	Malnutrition: 1,275,000

That's more than a million lives lost every year to unnecessary disease in the United States alone. If ever there was a situation befitting the phrase "room for growth," this is it; with proper nutrition, these lives lost to unnecessary or premature disease can be saved, and the enormous financial burden redirected toward funding projects and policies that improve our communities' well-being.

---

* Although these numbers are approximate, I have erred on the side of caution and provided conservative estimates. For instance, although nutrition can play a role in chronic lower respiratory disease, it would be very difficult to estimate a percentage of lives affected, so I have therefore chosen to leave that number as is. In the case of medical errors, I have made calculations using the lower estimate of deaths caused by medical errors (250,000, though estimates have been as high as 440,000).[34] Moreover, I have not even accounted for the many more preventable diseases not listed in the top six (perhaps the most notable of these is type II diabetes, which can be treated by nutrition in nearly 100 percent of cases).

If I am correct in this assessment, as the evidence suggests, then why are more people not focusing on nutrition as a solution? Why did my father, and so many others, not learn of Morrison's heart disease study, which was conducted well before my father's second, fatal heart attack? Why isn't nutrition fully embedded in the training and practice of cardiologists, oncologists, and other medical practitioners, from top to bottom? Why are we not more interested in learning from the dietary patterns of other cultures that show almost no incidence of heart disease,[35] our number one killer? Why do we continue to underplay nutrition's significance, and instead devote massive amounts of time and resources to invasive procedures and pharmaceutical Band-Aids?

Two fundamental observations help to answer these questions. The first is that the prevailing cultural narrative in our society tells us that malnutrition and disease are only partially connected. The extent to which people believe this depends on the disease (e.g., more people will say that nutrition plays a role in heart disease than cancer), but in general our society does not consider malnutrition to be the primary cause of most disease, and certainly not the preferred cure. Even in cases where we do admit nutrition's role, it is often secondary. For instance, you have probably at some point been advised to eat well in order to minimize the risk of developing a genetically determined disease. The notion that nutrition can do more than minimize such risk—that it can even eliminate it, and in many cases trump genetic determinism—is not widely accepted. We give lip service to nutrition by advising "heart-healthy diets" and the like, but these are discussed superficially and always in conjunction with other lifestyle choices like exercise.

Crucially, though, we are also confused about nutrition. This is the second fundamental observation: our prevailing cultural narrative tells us that *even if* nutrition and health are closely connected, we *still* aren't sure what the healthiest diet looks like.

For the rest of this chapter and the two that follow it, I will be focusing on the first of these observations: that (mal)nutrition is not fully appreciated as a determinant of disease and health. The second point—the confusion infecting our attitudes toward and uses for nutrition—will feature heavily in Parts II and III of this book. For now, though, it bears repeating that the

WFPB dietary lifestyle is controversial because it challenges *both* prevailing narratives in our society.

CANCER AS A CASE STUDY: THE NEVER-ENDING WAR

Nowhere is the power of nutrition, and its inverse, malnutrition, more underappreciated than in the field of cancer. It also happens to be the field to which I have devoted the majority of my research career, and so I can speak to the attitudes that pervade it with more authority than on any other field.

Consider, then, the following "Findings and Declaration of Purpose," copied and pasted from legislation[36] passed by the United States Congress. I like this example because it illustrates the failure of our disease-care system better than most:

(a) The Congress finds and declares:

> *(1) that the incidence of cancer is increasing and cancer is the disease which is the major health concern of Americans today;*
> *(2) that new scientific leads, if comprehensively and energetically exploited, may significantly advance the time when more adequate preventive and therapeutic capabilities are available to cope with cancer;*
> *(3) that cancer is a leading cause of death in the United States;*
> *(4) that the present state of our understanding of cancer is a consequence of broad advances across the full scope of the biomedical sciences;*
> *(5) that a great opportunity is offered as a result of recent advances in the knowledge of this dread disease to conduct energetically a national program against cancer;*
> *(6) that in order to provide for the most effective attack on cancer it is important to use all of the biomedical resources of the National Institutes of Health; and*
> *(7) that the programs of the research institutes which comprise the National Institutes of Health have made it possible to bring into being*

*the most productive scientific community centered upon health and
disease that the world has ever known.*

*(b) It is the purpose of this Act to enlarge the authorities of the National
Cancer Institute and the National Institutes of Health in order to advance
the national effort against cancer.*

You may understandably think this sounds like a good start. After all, who could argue against increased efforts against cancer, the coordinated effort and use of all the NIH, and the enlarged authority of institutions engaged in this critical fight? As this law observes, cancer is a leading cause of death, so these efforts seem apt and well timed.

At least, they seem apt and well timed until you realize that this legislation, the National Cancer Act, was not passed just recently. I'm sorry to have misled you, but I feel it proves a point. This bill was not passed this year or last, but all the way back in 1971, precisely between the passing of my mother-in-law and the passing of my father. It was passed in the same year that Nixon signed an amendment to lower the voting age to eighteen; a year when forty cents was enough to purchase a gallon of gas; the year when Apollo 14 was launched only a few months before the opening of a new theme park named Disney World.

Clearly, many things have changed in the nearly fifty years since Congress passed the National Cancer Act of 1971. But what concerns me most are the things that have *not* changed. Cancer remains a leading cause of death. Advances across all biomedical sciences continue to astound, and have contributed greatly to increasing "the present state of our understanding," but what benefits have we reaped from that understanding? Our ability to treat cancer has not improved, despite an extraordinary amount of resources dedicated to this mission. Last and most important, nutrition remains as undervalued and underutilized now as it was back then.

Hailed as the first strike in the "war on cancer," the National Cancer Act of 1971 is not the result of bad intentions, but of a faulty premise. It updated and retooled the National Cancer Institute to its current form, established new cancer research centers, and signaled a new, proactive campaign against one of our most dreaded diseases. The faulty premise undermining it—the flawed assumption that hasn't been proven out—is that the NCI and NIH were suitably armed for the war on cancer, when in fact their armory was and is missing the single most potent weapon in the war on cancer: nutrition. Among the twenty-seven institutes and centers at NIH, not a single one is dedicated to its study.

It's not just hopeful defenders of nutrition who would critique the war on cancer. Many established cancer professionals agree. In an article published in *The Lancet* a few years ago,[37] one critic characterized the war on cancer well: "Despite extraordinary progress in our understanding of disease pathogenesis, in most cases and for most forms of cancer this war has not been won." I'm sure you will agree with the author's most sobering concerns about cancer in the twenty-first century: (1) "cancer treatments are very expensive," (2) cancer treatments "[produce] only transitory clinical benefit," and (3) "the instrumental mutations and rearrangements of the human genome in the transformed cancer cells are extremely complex," and therefore extremely difficult to study.

Ultimately, however, the author does not demand a radical shift in strategy, and definitely not a prominent role for nutrition. Rather, he intensifies and doubles down on the war metaphor. He describes a "military battlespace" strategy capable of "incorporating information about the enemy's characteristics and armamentarium, precise topographical maps of all potential battlefields and war zones, the weather, and other environmental factors, along with a census of friendly forces and their capabilities, in all relevant geographical locations." In other, simpler words, he calls for a more sophisticated battle plan, but ultimately one that still relies on a technological understanding of cancer and medicine. The author does not discount the war on cancer's efforts, but instead argues for a more technically impressive application of what we have learned: "Although the dual metaphors of the war on cancer and of magic bullets to kill cancers *have been useful, now is the time to refine them*, factoring in extraordinary advances in knowledge about cancer science and medicine" (emphasis added). Rather than question the magic bullet premise, in which each specific disease can be combated by a specific drug, without side effects, he encourages us to invent a more perfect, more targeted magic bullet that does not hit anything other than its target. Assuming such a thing even exists (no small assumption), I wonder how long it will take to find it?

Meanwhile, the war has gone global. In another *Lancet* article, researchers Paolo Vineis and Christopher P. Wild[38] at the International Agency for Cancer Research (of the World Health Organization) make the case that "an increasing proportion of the [cancer] burden [is] falling on low-income and middle-income countries . . . urgent action is needed . . . [and that] primary prevention is the most effective way to fight cancer." I agree with all three of these statements. However, they refer only to strategies of primary prevention, whereas I would add that it is also time to consider the effect of this same nutrition protocol on cancer *treatment*. If our primary prevention strategies cannot integrate the strongest research findings on cancer, including those involving nutrition, then our organizational and structural interventions will never reach their full potential. The war on cancer will continue to amass an alarming body count and place tremendous demands on our resources and attention, only now on a global level.

I could critique the strategies of cancer researchers all day, but we must not forget about other branches of the biomedical establishment. If researchers specializing in disease are like strategists, holed up in their bunkers and studying the enemies' defenses, out on the field we have that valiant class of soldier we call Doctor. Understand, I am not blaming any individual here, but the system as a whole, and its disregard of nutrition. These soldiers are fighting a losing battle, because their weapons, their thoughts and actions, are limited. Given scalpels, pills, and radiation, they do not consider (or comprehend) strawberries, potatoes, and radicchio as agents of health.

And how could they? Not a single US medical school trains doctors in nutrition. Of the approximately 130 official medical specialties for which services can be reimbursed, nutrition isn't one of them. Doctors and nurses are the face of health care, responsible for delivering information and treatment to the public, yet they're given no financial reimbursement for nutritional services or education on the medical marvels of nutrition. It's as if they've been blindfolded, spun round and round, and asked to lead the way. Is it any surprise that they sometimes seem to be stumbling in the dark?

The failed war on cancer displays contemporary attitudes toward nutrition and disease better than any other example I can think of. As with the broader trends in our society's health, it illustrates a stubborn persistence that has not paid off. The incidence of cancer has declined somewhat in recent decades as a result of decreased smoking-related lung cancer, but overall we're losing the war. One might think that, faced with such a struggle, we would be more open to alternative approaches, but this has not been the case at all. Instead, we have seen nearly the opposite. Despite the impotence of conventional cancer prevention and treatment strategies, the medical establishment clings to them. Nutrition has received almost no attention, and any suggestion that it might deserve attention is regarded with skepticism.

To understand how nutrition came to be so underutilized, and why these attitudes persist today, it's helpful to examine the history of research into the relationship between nutrition and disease, especially cancer. It is in this history that key patterns emerge—patterns that continue to dominate our attitudes and practices, often beyond our awareness.

CHAPTER TWO

THE HIDDEN HISTORY OF NUTRITION AND DISEASE

Nothing is more responsible for the good old days than a bad memory.
—Franklin Pierce Adams

The episode I discussed in the introduction, the 1982 National Academy of Sciences (NAS) report on diet and cancer that I coauthored and the unusual opposition that followed, was a key moment in my career—not only because it shattered my naïveté and revealed how controversial dietary recommendations about protein could be, but also because it gave me many questions to explore in the years that followed. It encouraged

me to reflect on the role institutions play in the dissemination of information, the responsibility of dissident voices within institutions, and, in general,
the painful side effects of scientific advancement. Crucially, it also encouraged me to look deeper into the history of nutrition and disease research,
especially when it came to cancer.

Like others on the NAS committee, I had assumed that our findings on
the diet–nutrition–cancer association were relatively new, and that new ideas
in science naturally attract criticism. After all, most of the research cited in
our report was published in the 1960s and '70s. The earliest of all the research
papers we cited was published in 1931.[1] Still, I sensed that there might be
something more insidious in the reaction we had received, something worth
unpacking further. The supposed novelty of our report failed to explain the
degree of criticism we faced. It seemed to me that there was something more
to this story than new science versus old science. In fact, the criticism seemed
beyond intellect. It was visceral, intense, and clearly tethered to food industry
interests, especially those of animal-protein-based foods.

Eventually, I turned to the past for insight. I took a deep dive into
the history of nutrition and cancer, hoping to find some greater sense of
context—additional vantage points from which to consider the vitriol I'd
experienced, both personally and professionally. I had the perfect opportunity to do just that when I spent a year at Oxford University on sabbatical
from 1985 to 1986. The year I spent there could not have come at a better
time. As I dug deeper into the history, I tried as much as possible to read
original manuscripts and reports. Consequently, I lived most of that year
in four libraries: the Bodleian Library and the Wellcome Trust Library in
Oxford, and the Royal College of Surgeons and Royal College of Physicians
in London.

Because I was unsure of where and when the disciplines of cancer and
nutrition may have previously overlapped, if ever, the little I did know could
be described, at best, as superficial. Thankfully, it didn't take long to find
a starting place: Frederick Hoffman's *Cancer and Diet* (1937),[2] brought
to my attention by a postdoctoral resident in my Cornell laboratory, Tom
O'Connor.*

---

* Now a senior professor at University College Cork in Ireland.

HOFFMAN: A HIDDEN PIONEER

Hoffman was an author I had never heard of before, and what I found in *Cancer and Diet* was exceptional: a 749-page book with a vast number of references investigating the possibility of a nutrition–cancer association. To my surprise, it quickly and definitively proved to me that our 1982 NAS report was not especially new and that research into nutrition and cancer had once overlapped. In my initial scan of the book, I was especially impressed by Hoffman's exhaustiveness. In his own words, "every work referred to, otherwise than in abstract, has been read carefully by myself from beginning to end to make sure that no important observation should be missed." He goes on to say that his review[2] is limited to approximately 200 authorities because he had "neither the strength nor the time to visit other libraries for the purpose of amplification and completeness."*

Reading this was an eye-opener, to say the least. *Limited* to 200 authorities? The science supporting the conclusions of the 1982 NAS committee was surprisingly deeper, perhaps far richer, than we'd thought. Contained within that realization was, I believe, a valuable lesson and warning about the nature of science. Too often, "trailblazers" of the day fail to investigate the full breadth of the scientific literature. They assume, often smugly, that their discoveries are uniquely novel. Our NAS committee was guilty of this, too. We assumed that our survey of past literature was relatively comprehensive, when in fact we barely scratched the surface.

Hoffman's *Cancer and Diet* proved to be an invaluable resource, both for its exhaustive content and for its professional presentation, but it also raised many questions. Chiefly, who was Frederick Hoffman and why had I never heard of him before? He died in 1946, only thirty-five years before our 1982 report, yet he was a complete mystery to me. The more I learned about his work, the more perplexed I was by his erasure. He was by any measure one of the most productive and professional scientists I have ever encountered, yet it was very difficult to find details about his life—though I did find at least one other author, Francis Sypher, who in a 2012 journal

---

* Hoffman had been suffering from Parkinson's disease for about ten years when he wrote his 1937 book.

article asks similar questions about why Hoffman was so abruptly forgotten when he died.[3]

What few biographical details do persist can be summarized quickly.[3] Hoffman arrived in the United States from Germany in 1884. He had a restless youth and certainly didn't come from wealth. In fact, he was unable to afford secondary school, and he never attended university. In his early years, he had a yen for traveling the world and learning new things. Perhaps in order to maintain that lifestyle, he worked on an assortment of odd jobs, until he finally landed a more permanent position with the Prudential Insurance Company in Newark, New Jersey, where he worked for the next forty years. Despite his lack of formal education, his aptitude for statistics made him an ideal candidate for actuarial work, including calculating and predicting disease risk. He was apparently quite good at this; so good, in fact, that he was able to ascend into the higher echelons of professional statistics and eventually become president of the American Statistical Association.[4]

In these biographical details, we get perhaps the first glimpse of why he has not been celebrated in the histories of cancer research. His poor immigrant upbringing, missing as it did a typical education, squares with his later outsider status. What's extraordinary, though, is how far he went despite that combination of obstacles. His work ethic is hard to deny, and his productive output was surely enough to rival even the most privileged researchers of his day. Throughout his career, he published "1300 items, including 28 major works of 100 or more pages," according to Sypher.[3] Early in his career, he was especially interested in the effects of the "dusty trades" industry[4] (a term used to describe occupations in which workers were exposed to heavy amounts of dust, including sand blasters, graphite miners, and carpet mill workers) on respiratory problems like tuberculosis and "dust phthisis in the granite stone industry."[3] His work in this area had a significant impact on labor legislation affecting occupational hazards.[5] As such, he was a charter member of the National Tuberculosis Association.[4]

But it was cancer that dominated his focus, especially at the peak of his career. On this topic alone, he authored sixteen books and an estimated one hundred professional publications.[5] His early interest was in trying to understand why cancer rates had increased so much since the beginning of the 1900s and why cancer rates varied so much both within the US[6] and internationally.[7] In 1915, he published an 826-page tome that tackled this question directly, documenting the great range of cancer rates in different parts of the world.[7] Eight years later, he studied cancer death rates, controlled for age, in twenty-two cities and localities in the US and elsewhere.[6] One of the most interesting details of this study, from my perspective, is that he surveyed consumption of various food groups, including "green vegetables, fresh fruits, cereals, white bread, condensed and conserved food, meat, sugar, salt, etc."

Another striking biographical detail, given his later obscurity, was Hoffman's very central role in founding the American Cancer Society (ACS; founded as the American Society for the Control of Cancer). In 1913, he delivered a much anticipated speech to the American Gynecological Society titled "The Menace of Cancer," in which he expressed alarm at rising cancer rates.[8] This speech led directly to the founding of the ACS, as the organization itself acknowledges in a picture in a lobby showcase in their Atlanta headquarters. In that speech, he recommended that "the nutritional influences on the induction of cancer be analyzed." He also called for greater proactivity: "The time has come for a nationwide interest in the problem of prevention and control [of cancer]." In *Cancer and Diet*, published twenty-four years later, he took an even firmer stance on nutrition's role in cancer. The evidence by that time was, he said, "fully sufficient to prove that cancer from the earliest times has been looked upon as a question involving dietary and nutritional considerations."[2]

If such bold assertions about the connection between nutrition and cancer come as a surprise to you, you're not alone. For decades, the status quo in cancer research and treatment has followed the exact opposite line of thinking. From the earliest times that I had studied, prior to my discovery of Hoffman, cancer was not looked upon as a question involving dietary and nutritional considerations. Rather, since the beginning of my career, and certainly now, cancer has been seen as a question involving *genetic* considerations, with discourse centering on mutation-causing environmental toxins (mutagens)—which fits the presumption that cancer is caused by specific agents acting locally. (I will have much to say about local theories of cancer in the coming pages.) Likewise, local treatment protocols have been completely dominant. The notion that dietary and nutritional considerations are relevant to the development or treatment of cancer is so far removed from existing thinking that many professionals, then and now, reject it out of hand. And yet here was a seemingly authoritative figure—a central figure in the formation of the ACS!—claiming the opposite. Clearly something had changed.

Again, I wondered, why have we not heard this information? The fact that Hoffman, by many accounts, was so involved in the formation of the ACS suggests to me that his story is far more than that of a forgotten statistician. It's easy to understand how a brilliant but less visible professional figure might be forgotten over time. Surely this is a common occurrence. But in Hoffman's case, he *was* visible—visible enough even to give what many regarded as the organization's founding speech. He was indeed a forgotten statistician, but also an abandoned leader. His call for increased research on the role of nutrition in cancer, his warnings, and his evidence were all neglected, as if by mandate.

Perhaps you think Hoffman's obscurity can be explained another way. Maybe his ideas were already outdated by the 1980s, when those of us on the NAS committee surveyed the literature on cancer and nutrition? Perhaps they are even more outdated now? Maybe his findings simply could not stand the test of time, and were later proved wrong? These are good hypothetical questions, but again they do not match the historical evidence. Take a closer look and you will see that many of his observations have aged well. Some even seem downright prophetic.

Hoffman's massive 1915 study of cancer mortality rates[7] is surely a classic. It cites 579 sources and includes a meticulous presentation of statistical methodology and conclusions in its first 221 pages. There he provides critical commentary on the importance of using age-standardized data, a method of adjusting data to account for differences in the distribution of ages of populations now widely accepted as necessary when conducting epidemiological research. Although impressive in its own right, this study also formed the basis for the first United States Cancer Census.[9] In other words, far from fading into irrelevance, Hoffman's work here set the foundation for future progress in the field.

In 1923, he organized the San Francisco Cancer Survey, which went on to publish nine reports over the next eleven years.[6] It was in this survey that he first analyzed the effects of tobacco and eventually concluded that "the increase in cancer of the lungs observed in this and many other countries is, in all probability, to a certain extent directly traceable to the more common practice of cigarette smoking and the inhalation of cigarette smoke. The latter practice unquestionably increases the danger of cancer development."[10] He also warned against the growing trend of cigarette smoking by women. Of course, these observations are obvious to us now, but Hoffman's findings came *twenty years before* the classic studies on smoking and lung cancer published by Wynder and Graham[11] and Doll and Hill,[12] *thirty-three years before* the US Surgeon General's report on smoking,[13] and *more than fifty years before* the debates on smoking and lung cancer still taking place in the mid-'80s, when I was first discovering Hoffman's work. When I asked Sir Richard Doll, the famous Oxford epidemiologist who was rightfully nominated for the Nobel Prize several times for his discovery of the link between tobacco smoking and lung cancer in the 1950s, if he knew of Hoffman's work in the '30s, he could not initially recall. After some reminding, he did remember Hoffman, but only as "that insurance man"—another example of how scientists (myself included, at times!) often don't do a very good job of recording and recalling the findings of those who preceded us, and sometimes fail to appreciate other points of view when they do not originate from established scientific institutions. Nonetheless, Hoffman's work has aged exceptionally well. That is not to say that his findings were not controversial, but that perhaps he was ahead of his time.

And what did he have to say about cancer and diet? His position was unequivocal: "excessive nutrition" is either cancer's "chief cause" or "at least a contributory factor of the first importance." By excessive nutrition, he meant the overconsumption of rich foods found in industrialized nations, particularly meat.

When I read Hoffman's book, I had already been an experimental researcher on these topics for over twenty years, and so I was fascinated to discover in his work many of the same things I had observed in my own research, anathema though they were to the medical establishment. But my first reaction to these parallels was not glee or gratification. No, as a scientist, I was ashamed—that this information was published as recently as 1937, and reviewed such a long and revealing history of research efforts, yet I had never heard it. I was confused and concerned, but mainly ashamed of what seemed to me a vast and collective amnesia. Few individuals, if any, contributed more than Hoffman to our knowledge on cancer causation during the years 1913 to 1937. And yet you wouldn't know it. Today, I cannot find even a single reference to his paper on smoking[10] or to his monumental 1937 book on diet and cancer.[2]

The cancer research barons of the period were apparently willing to let him collect data for a cancer census, but not interpret the data he'd collected. H. T. Deelman, professor of pathology at the University of Gröningen, the Netherlands, acknowledged Hoffman's 1915 cancer atlas as "good and very serviceable" at the 1926 American Cancer Society conference at Lake Mohonk, but then attacked Hoffman's right to interpret the data. According to Deelman, Hoffman had overstepped his role as a statistician when he "arrogated to himself the part of cancer investigator."[14] At the same ACS conference, he reiterated the skepticism of British tumor transplant* researcher Ernest Bashford,[15] who suggested that statistics on varying cancer rates around the world, like those cited by Hoffman, were not to be trusted. (Bashford claimed that statistics on cancer incidence from Ireland were less precise than those from England, and that statistics from poorer countries were even less precise, though I never found any compelling evidence to support this speculative dismissal.) In short, Deelman denied any connection whatsoever between cancer and diet. He dismissed the work of Hoffman and others out of hand, describing their conclusions as "specious statements." And to them, he exclaimed: "Bring proof of what you are writing!" An ironic suggestion, I think, given that (1) he was unwilling to consider the statistics already provided and (2) his targets were consistently excluded from such conferences.

What threat did Hoffman and other researchers of nutrition and cancer pose? I can think of many possibilities, based on similar backlash I have received throughout my career. Did their views threaten the market for surgical services, as mine have sometimes done?[16,17] Did their views, tending toward vegetarianism (though not always explicitly supporting the label[2]), upset social norms and make them seem timid and effeminate? Is it possible

---

* In these studies, tumor tissue was transplanted from one animal to another to see if it would grow.

that diet, nutrition, and cancer reports were ignored and vilified because surgeons and other medical men simply could not comprehend a complex nutritional issue for which they had no training?

On Hoffman specifically, did his conclusion that "the principal dietary errors of the present day consist of a too heavy intake of protein and . . . sugar," in the Eighth Annual Report of his San Francisco Survey,[6] anger the relevant food industries? Might his views on other topics have contributed? He spoke and published on a wide range of controversial topics, including birth control,[18] public health policy,[19,20] national health insurance,[21] race,[4,5] and workplace legislation.[21–25] Did he personally irritate his peers by discussing some of these issues?* Did he threaten the establishment's preferred method for communicating with the public and therefore undermine the role of institutions such as the ACS[26,27] and the British Empire Cancer Campaign (BECC)?[28–30] George Soper, ACS managing director, was very clear[31,32] in how he viewed the role of cancer institutions: he believed they should be developed, managed, and informed only by physicians, especially surgeons, who should serve as the primary (if not only) source of public information on cancer.† Was Hoffman's work dismissed because he wasn't beholden to any medical institution? Although this gave him greater freedom to explore hypotheses wherever they might lead, did his outsider status also limit those institutions' respect for him?

Do similar questions apply to cancer research and health care as a whole in the twenty-first century?

I don't mean to suggest that Hoffman was without fault; it would be a dangerous mistake to make an idol of him. Nevertheless, he does provide an excellent foil for both the cancer researchers of his day and more recent ones. Unlike many of his colleagues, he didn't arrive to the field of cancer

---

* Some of his earliest work concerning mortality trends among African Americans was critiqued, but there's no contemporary indication that this work contributed to his ostracism, or that it had anything to do with his work on cancer.

† The reasoning behind this is clear. In the words of Howard Lilienthal: "The physician belongs to that enlightened class which, in principal at least, believes in the efficacy of the early and radical extirpation of malignant growths"[33] (as opposed to alternatives, such as nutrition). In Britain, another cancer specialist even claimed that propaganda would play some role in the control of cancer.[34]

research with preconceived ideas about nutrition. On numerous occasions, he was very careful not to overextend his views. Rather than claiming proof, he nearly always encouraged further study. In the large case-control study he began in 1924[35] and reported in 1937,[2] he concluded that he had found no evidence to support an effect of eating meat on cancer risk. This isn't proof of him defending meat intake, but simply of him being a competent scientist. About 99 percent of the cases and controls in that study ate meat, thus limiting any conclusions he could have made in either direction. In some cases, he may have been exceedingly conservative. In 1925,[36] he recommended that contemporary treatment procedures of surgery, radiotherapy, and early diagnosis were the best available methods of cancer control. This conclusion was based on the existing data supporting those procedures (data that were deeply flawed in many ways, as I will discuss in chapter three). Yet, unlike most of his colleagues, he wasn't afraid to reevaluate his own views and even the usefulness of statistics in certain cases. In 1927, he began to waver in his support of the use of cancer survival data to evaluate treatment. When studying statistics from Mexico,[37] he was "inclined to think that errors are more common in which non-malignant tumors are diagnosed as malignant than otherwise."

If not for their forgetfulness, what would the cancer research establishment of today make of Hoffman? What would they make of his willingness to adopt new perspectives, never leap to conclusions, and generally keep an open mind? Is there something about that flexibility that is fundamentally incompatible with the mentality that has come to dominate the field? Here is another reason why we should not make an idol of Hoffman: these traits—flexibility, open-mindedness, and vigilance—are merely proof of a competent scientist. They require no genius or sainthood. They should be the standards to which we hold *all* of our researchers. A world in which flexibility and open-mindedness are exceptions rather than rules is not a fertile breeding ground for truth.

For that matter, what would the cancer research establishment of today make of Hoffman's peers and predecessors?

THE COMPANY YOU KEEP, OR DISCARD

As I dug deeper into this history, I tried as much as possible to read the work Hoffman referenced. As a result, I came to discover a wide and fascinating cast of other historical characters wrestling with questions similar to my own about nutrition and cancer. That these questions were apparently off limits by the time I "came of age," forbidden enough that simply raising them threatened to undermine my reputation among my peers, suggests that the discourse surrounding cancer and nutrition research had become more limited since the years of Hoffman and his peers. The discourse then was not utopic either. There were certainly issues of professional reputation, real or imagined, affecting what Hoffman was or was not allowed to say throughout the era I surveyed, and there is no denying that he ran up against many boundaries. But well before Hoffman, especially during the nineteenth century, there was at least a more open, rich, and vibrant interchange of controversial information.

Throughout the two hundred years of literature that Hoffman reviewed, many foods were accused of contributing to the prevalence of cancer. However, the prevailing recommendation was to avoid "overnutrition" (synonymous with the "excessive nutrition" that Hoffman warned against). Overnutrition was not characterized by caloric excess alone, but also by the type of food being consumed in excess. On individual food groups, the most common recommendations were those against meat consumption and those encouraging more vegetable and fruit consumption. According to Hoffman, protein was the first and most frequent individual nutrient associated with overnutrition. On this last point, Hoffman refers to William Lambe and the early years of the nineteenth century.

William Lambe was a Fellow of the Royal College of Physicians in London. Both in 1809[38] and 1815,[39] he warned "against the danger of excess in food consumption, particularly meat and other protein products."*[f] Twice he proposed to study the effect of the "vegetable diet" on breast cancer patients

---

* This verbatim comment cited both by W. Roger Williams (see page 44) in 1908 and Hoffman may have been a paraphrase of Lambe's very strong views against meat consumption, as I could not locate it in either of Lambe's books. It is, however, an accurate representation of his views published elsewhere.

at the famed Middlesex Hospital in London, and twice his colleagues turned him down.[40] Accounts suggest that they considered Lambe a crank and that his advocacy of meatless diets (the word "vegetarian" did not enter the nomenclature until the middle of the nineteenth century) drew great scorn from many, including the cancer surgeons at Middlesex[40] who denied his study proposals. Lambe was thus an important figure, and a forerunner of later researchers into the association between cancer and nutrition, but far too ostracized to ever achieve his full potential.

But that doesn't mean his recommendations were without support or application. Indeed, one of his highly respected contemporaries, John Abernethy, recommended that "the powers of the [dietary] regimen recommended by Dr. Lambe should be fairly tried." In his own words, Dr. Lambe had suffered "ill health and ailments" until age eighteen. At that point, he "finally" undertook (in February 1806) "what he had been contemplating for some time—to abandon animal food altogether and everything analagous to it, and to continue to confine himself wholly to vegetable food." He wrote that he "never found the smallest real ill consequence from this change . . . and sank neither in strength, flesh, nor in spirits."[41] According to another friend and colleague, Lambe at seventy-two years of age was

> very gentlemanly in manners and venerable in appearance . . . He told me . . . that his health was better now than at forty . . . [and] he considers himself as likely to live thirty years longer as to have lived to his present age . . . Although he is seventy-two years of age he walks into town, a distance of three miles from his residence, every morning and back at night.[41]

Personal life aside, Lambe later "began to use his diet as a cure for patients ill with cancer," a practice that Abernethy once again supported. Abernethy reasoned "that the body can be perfectly nourished by vegetables," that "all great changes of the constitution are more likely to be effected by alterations of diet and modes of life than by medicine," and that Lambe's diet offered "a source of hope and consolation to the patient in a disease in which medicine is known to be unavailing and in which surgery affords no more than a temporary relief." Still, despite this support from the renowned Abernethy, Lambe's colleagues twice denied his research proposals.*

In Hoffman's opinion,[2] it was not Lambe but John Hughes Bennett in 1849 who provided "the first definite indication of the recognition of cancer as a nutritional disease." Bennett was a senior professor of clinical medicine at the University of Edinburgh, where he studied the relationship between cancer and body fat. On that relationship, he said, "an excessive cell development (as in cancer) must materially be modified by diminishing the amount of fatty elements, which originally furnish elementary granules and nuclei; the circumstances which diminish obesity, and a tendency to the formation of fat, would seem *a priori* to be opposed to the cancerous tendency."[42] In much simpler words, behavior that reduces the formation of fat (including diet) *should* lower the risk of cancerous growth. In 1865,[43] he remained convinced that tumor growth was associated with an "excess of nutrition" and added a more specific recommendation: "in carcinoma . . . the body . . . is for the most part fatty, and a diminution of this element in the food should be aimed at." On these points, modern-day evidence backs him up; there is considerable evidence linking obesity and cancer. Of course, not all of his assertions were bulletproof. His suggestion that reduced fat consumption necessarily controls levels of body fat is an oversimplification, given modern evidence.

In the postscript to his book in 1849,[42] Bennett recommended an 1845 book by George MacIlwain,[44] yet another researcher and physician who

---

* Now, after more than 200 years, Lambe's proposed trial on breast cancer patients is finally underway. My son Tom and his wife, Erin, both physicians, are at last conducting a professionally approved research study on stage IV breast cancer patients. This new study was approved after careful Institutional Review Board scrutiny by his institution, the University of Rochester Medical Center. Receiving that approval was neither quick nor easy. There remains profound doubt in the professional cancer community that nutrition, provided by a "vegetable diet," as Lambe called it, could have anything to do with cancer, especially as a possible treatment. The conditions required by the review board for this new proposal—limiting the testing of the whole food, plant-based (WFPB) diet only as an adjunct to traditional pharmacologic treatment instead of testing it alone—illustrate the medical establishment's cautious paternalism. Even for individuals who would elect to use the WFPB diet alone, medical authorities insist on the concurrent use of "proven" chemotherapy drugs. Never mind that the effectiveness of these drugs ranges from highly questionable to unproven.

linked cancer with dietary excesses and warned strongly against "grease, fat, and alcohol" because of their toxic effects on the liver. MacIlwain further observed that "of the cause of [cancer], I am at least certain of this, that either the food contains something unusual, or that some of the assimilating organs are acting on it in some unusual manner, or both. This seems indisputable." What makes MacIlwain unique from my perspective is that he considered the broader effects of the whole diet on cancer, rather than only specific nutrients. There's little doubt that he would have shared many of Bennett's concerns about dietary fat, but his focus was not nearly as singular.

As the decades passed, this lineage of medical authorities speaking out about diet's role in cancer showed no sign of fading. John Shaw, of the Royal College of Surgeons, England, recommended in 1907[45] increased consumption of vegetable foods and decreased use of animal foods, alcohol, tea, tobacco, and drugs for controlling cancer. And just one year later, W. Roger Williams, member of the Royal College of Surgeons in London, published an extensive book on the history of cancer arguing that nutrition should have a central role in cancer research. According to Hoffman, this book should have been a classic in the field: "[marking] an epoch in cancer literature, reviewing the whole subject with absolute impartiality and resulting in a cancer classic of the first importance."

According to Williams's text, "probably no single factor is more potent in determining the outbreak of cancer in the predisposed, than excessive feeding." This concern for excess should by now be a familiar one. To elaborate this point, Williams targets the "gluttonous consumption of proteids—especially meat—which is such a characteristic of this age," insufficient vegetable intake, and sedentary lifestyles as other contributing factors. (I wonder, what would Williams make of our meat consumption now, more than a century later, and of our amplified gluttony?)

One last point of interest in Williams's book is his emphasis on the environmental origin of cancer and the effects of migration on cancer risk. The uneven distribution of disease throughout the US and world was also a subject that fascinated Hoffman. Combined with research on migration (mentioned in chapter one), uneven distribution of disease suggests that cancer is related to lifestyle factors (also said to be "environmental"). Similar views were expressed much earlier, in 1846, by another eminent physician and researcher, Walter Hayle Walshe,[46] who presented cancer mortality data to show that it was primarily a disease of "civilization."

RESURRECTING THE VOICELESS

I could surely devote an entire book to these individuals and their greatest works, but I think I have made my point: there is a very long tradition of investigating and believing in a role for nutrition in the formation of cancer (and indeed, disease more generally). If progress in this field has been slow, as the allegation often goes, then it is for neither lack of effort nor lack of interest, at least on the part of certain groups of scientists. There have, however, been many impediments, as seen with Lambe, whose proposals to study the effect of diet on cancer were denied by his surgeon colleagues; with the forgotten Hoffman; and well beyond. Those authorities who bemoan a lack of convincing evidence on these issues are often the same ones who both ignore and impede, especially proactively, the flow of the ample evidence that does exist. I am not suggesting this as a full-blown conspiracy, but as a historical fact.

There are many other figures from this period whose research I could cite. My own, albeit incomplete, review of the early literature suggests that Hoffman's *Cancer and Diet* captured only a fraction of the discourse surrounding nutrition and cancer (perhaps 20–30 percent). Nevertheless, many of these findings are uniquely perceptive in light of modern evidence. Here are a few gems:

- John Howard in 1811,[47] fellow of the Royal College of Surgeons and author of practical observations on cancer, and many other writers in the next 175 years (including extensive comments by W. B. Thomson in 1932[48]), argued that constipation was an important predictor of cancer. Howard came to this view after forty years of practice with cancer patients. The consensus then, as it is now, was that plant foods prevent constipation. This association of colon cancer and other Western diseases with constipation has for many years been attributed to insufficient consumption of dietary fiber, a nutritional component only found in plants, as reviewed by Dennis Burkitt in 1975.[49]

- John Hughes Bennett in 1849[42] recommended that nutrition standards should reflect both upper and lower limits, saying, "In the one case, we should do all we can to bring the nutrition up to and above the average (to reduce the risk of tuberculosis); in the other, down to and below it (to reduce the risk of cancer)."

- J. Braithwaite in 1901[50] suggested that three of the principal causes of cancer were salt, high nourishment (especially meat), and "old cells with effete [ineffectual] nourishment."

- Francis Hare in 1905[51] described an "old standing idea in the profession that the increase of malignant disease is in some way associated with the increased cheapness and improved quality of the world's food supply." *An old standing idea . . . in 1905?*

- In 1908,[52] the aforementioned Roger Williams demonstrated a parallel relationship between "good nutrition" of the day (that is, an affluent diet including more meat) and cancer, heart disease, diabetes, arthritis, and gallstones.

- Thomson in 1932[48] claimed that "food is undoubtedly of great importance in the study of cancer." *Undoubtedly of great importance . . . in 1932?* He also worried that "many surgeons, radiologists, and chemotherapists scoff at the idea of food exerting any influence in the cause, arrest, or cure of the disease, and they carry their conviction so far as to put their patients on ordinary fare as soon as possible after an operation and also during treatment by radiation." On this point, almost nothing has changed. Cancer professionals continue to ignore a nutritional effect, relying heavily on surgery, radiology, and chemotherapy, and we often hear about hospital patients being given "ordinary fare" following operations.

It bears emphasizing that just as our 1982 NAS report was but one part of a much larger procession, so too were these nineteenth- and twentieth-century cancer professionals. The literature on diet, nutrition, and cancer goes back far earlier than most contemporary readers would think, at least to ancient Greece[53] and China;[54] it certainly was a surprise to me. Hare was absolutely correct when he suggested that the nutrition–cancer link was an old standing idea. We have only forgotten this old wisdom.

In the 1980s when I was discovering this work, and certainly still today, the predominant belief was that cancer is a genetic disease for which nutrition can do little. Similar attitudes also pervade our study and treatment of other lifestyle-related diseases, as I discussed in the previous chapter. But all the way back in 1676, Richard Wiseman[55] concluded that cancer "might arise from an errour [sic] in Diet, a great acrimony* in the meats and drinks meeting with a fault in the first Concoction,† which, not being afterwards corrected in the Guts, suffers this acrimonious matter to ascend into the bloud [sic]." His preferred cure? To perform an exact "regulation in diet and way of living, advising to abstain from such salt, sharp and gross meats, as may dispose the bloud [sic] to acrimony." That's right—doctors have been calling for dietary interventions in the prevention and even *treatment* of cancer for more than 350 years! But who remembers their voices?

To return to the central theme of Part I, and add a new wrinkle, the WFPB diet is controversial because it challenges conventional attitudes and prevailing narratives about the causes and treatments of disease. Yet clearly these attitudes have not always been conventional and those narratives not always prevailing. Although the many historical figures cited in this chapter did not advocate for the WFPB diet exactly as I do, the general message is consistent: the food we eat *does* matter, including when it comes to cancer, and certain foods (especially foods containing animal protein) are especially harmful in that respect. The process by which this concept came to be forbidden deserves greater attention and raises many questions:

- How is history recorded and preserved in the sciences?
- What efforts have been made to study that history?
- How is discourse shaped in the sciences, and has this process changed over time?
- How are research questions and approved methods of study subsequently shaped by discourse?

---

* Biting sharpness to the taste or other bodily sense, pungency; irritancy; acridity.
† Digestion (of food) in the stomach and intestines.

•   How do research results reach the public?

The more I gave these and other questions my attention, the more I found that our practiced forgetfulness could be traced to the founding of cancer institutions, which have a tremendous power to shape all of the above—history, education, discourse, research questions, acceptable methods, communication with the public, and more.

CHAPTER THREE
DISEASE CARE
INSTITUTIONALIZED

Philosophy is not a theory but an activity.
—Ludwig Wittgenstein

That so many past commentators have acknowledged nutrition as an important factor in causing cancer is an important and revealing insight, but it only takes us so far. Clearly this acknowledgment of the nutrition–cancer link no longer jibes with the contemporary research and treatment of cancer, or indeed most other diseases commonly found in economically developed countries, and so the question remains: What changed?

To explain why advocates of nutrition have been ignored, we must take a more nuanced look at the early debates surrounding nutrition and other competing practices. What we discover in those debates is one question, above all others, that influenced the acceptance or rejection of nutrition's role: *Is cancer a local or a constitutional disease?* From the earliest times, cancer

49

professionals wrestled with this question, for it determined every aspect of their approach, from prevention to treatment, and from what experimental research was done to education and public policy making.

To define these terms, a *local* disease is one that attacks a particular part of the body and has a specific cause, and therefore can be dealt with precisely. *Particularity*, *specificity*, and *precision* are the key words here. Early proponents of the local theory of cancer believed that cancer was caused by isolated and identifiable agents such as wounds, bacteria, parasites, and viruses. (Today, cancer researchers who focus on single gene mutations or single environmental toxins are reflecting these same principles.) The corollary of that belief was that cancer could be locally (and simply) treated. In the earliest days of this debate, "local" treatment meant surgery. It's easy to understand how this theory became popular. Surgeons occupy positions of prestige and power, and the simplicity of the theory appeals to our rational minds. It translates well to both diagnosing a disease ("this cancer is of the breast, and it is caused by that specific agent") and prescribing a treatment ("remove the breast, remove the cancer").

On the other hand, the *constitutional* theory of cancer proposes that the disease has deeper origins, likely involving the complex pathways of metabolism that characterize nutrition's function.[1,2] Compared to the local theory's reliance on specific cancerous agents, the constitutional theory suggests more elusive causes. Far from the wounds, bacteria, parasites, or viruses credited by local-theory advocates, early proponents of the constitutional theory even suggested the possibility of *multiple* factors.[3-5] Suggestions that cancer might be multifactorial appeared in numerous publications:

- In 1888, the aforementioned W. Roger Williams (chapter two) cited British surgeon Campbell De Morgan, who observed that no matter how many clay pipe smokers get cancer of the lip or chimney sweeps get scrotal cancer, the "majority will not become cancerous, irritate how you will."[6] Ironically, De Morgan favored the local theory, but his statement here and Williams's interpretation certainly suggest the possibility of less visible factors, or perhaps even a combination of factors, in the cases of lip and scrotal cancer.

- In 1924, physician J. E. Barker hypothesized that cancer was caused by vitamin deficiency,[7] to which another doctor, Andrea Rabagliati,[3] responded that total diet played the greater part. (By virtue of the fact that nutrition a short while later was found to comprise multiple complex vitamins and other factors working in synchrony, any suggestion that nutrition plays a role in cancer is an argument for multifactorial causes, and supports the constitutional theory of disease.)
- In both 1907[8] and 1912,[4] R. Russell emphasized the multiple causes of cancer. Although he listed the consumption of animal flesh as one of those main causes, he also had the insight to warn that "animal flesh by itself without other stimulants does not appear of necessity to cause much cancer."[8]

On this final point, both my own experimental findings and the evidence of others tend to agree with Russell. The correlation between animal protein consumption and cancer risk is very strong, but the equation is not so elementary as animal protein = disease. (Sometimes people argue against this straw man, but it is not an honest representation of my own interpretation.) Instead, there are both direct and indirect effects on cancer from consuming animal protein. One indirect effect is that the more animal-based foods one eats, the less one consumes cancer-preventive plant-based foods packed with antioxidants, fiber, and other protective nutrients.[9] Recall the comment on nutrient composition in the Introduction, replicated here, which illustrates this point well. In particular, note the virtual exclusion of crucially important antioxidants, complex carbohydrates, and vitamins from animal foods (excepting small amounts of antioxidants and vitamins sometimes found in tissues of animals having recently consumed plant foods):

NUTRIENT COMPOSITIONS*

COMPONENT	PLANT	ANIMAL
Antioxidants	Only Made By Plants	Almost None
Complex Carbs	Only Made By Plants	None
Vitamins	Made By Plants	Almost None
Fat	~9–11%	~15–20%
Protein	~9–11%	~15–20%

PROCESSED FOODS are varied, likely worse

Unlike the surgical approach that advocates of the local theory champion, nutrition is a vastly intricate and interconnected process. Those who vouch for its role in causing or preventing cancer are *by necessity* considering multiple factors. This is evident in the greater nuance (and even uncertainty) expressed in early commentary. According to Frederick Hoffman,[10] physician Lucius Duncan Bulkley recognized nutrition's role in cancer causation in 1921,[11] but not without cautioning that "to understand and rightly treat the systemic condition belonging to cancer, which is indeed its basic factor, one needs to take a very broad view of the complex processes which pertain to metabolism and nutrition." Hoffman himself, in 1923,[12] questioned "if a single 'cause' will be found responsible for cancerous affections, for it would seem much more likely that a multitude of conditioning circumstances are responsible." He restated this view in 1924,[13] 1933,[14] and 1937.[10] Hoffman also references Bernhard Fischer-Wasels, director of the Pathological Institute of the University of Frankfurt, who emphasized the complexity of nutrition in 1935. The aforementioned Williams also recognized the importance of multiple factors.[15] In 1908, he argued against the notion of simple solutions (e.g., the chemotherapy marketed at the time) when given such complex biological problems. And of course, the "excessive" nutrition about which he wrote so much included countless nutrients interacting in a highly complex causal pathway.

What we see in the history, then, are two mostly incompatible theories. However, these theories are not incompatible on *all* levels. For example, it would be possible to view cancer as a constitutional disease but still deal with the crisis of a tumor by performing surgery, especially when there is sufficient evidence that the cancer being removed is self-contained, as in so-called benign or nonmetastatic tumors. The difference is in how one views the cause of that disease, and how one proceeds following that surgery. Those who vouched for the local theory focused on avoiding specific cancer-causing forces in the environment, whether a toxic chemical (poison), a virus, or a wound, and counted a removed tumor as a victory against that cancer. They did *not* consider nutrition to be an important part of cancer prevention or treatment. Conversely, those who vouched for the constitutional theory would also want to avoid toxins and viruses in the environment, for a host of other reasons not related to cancer alone, but would also follow up surgery with strategies to address what they viewed as the underlying causes of cancer, like nutrition.

Where these two theories become more incompatible is in a complete adoption of the constitutional theory, for that largely decreases the need for any local treatment protocols. Likewise, the complete adoption of the local theory leaves little room for constitutional treatment protocols, even as a supplemental measure. Just as the complete adoption of the constitutional theory questions the need for local treatment protocols, the complete adoption of the local theory decreases our focus on constitutional origins and treatments of disease. By confining cancer professionals to only one of these perspectives, we effectively limit the breadth and variety of treatment options available, to the great detriment of the public.

THE LOCAL THEORY PREVAILS

These two theories of cancer causation battled for well over a century, and certainly longer if you consider the competing, underlying beliefs and assumptions of each position. As early as 1784, Benjamin Bell of Edinburgh argued that breast cancer is a local disease, best cured by surgery.[16] In 1816, physician John Abernethy disagreed, as did William Lambe[17,18] and John Howard[19] during the same decade. Abernethy suggested that "the best timed and best conducted operation brings with it nothing but disgrace if the diseased propensities of the constitution are active and powerful."[2]

A couple decades later, at an 1844 French Academy of Medicine surgeons' conference in Paris, J. H. Bennett[20] reported that French physician Jean Cruveilhier was in a minority when he restated this view: "Cancer always depended upon a constitutional disorder, that local disease was the effect and not the cause, and to remove the first, while the latter was allowed to remain, was an irrational practice." But as you might expect, surgeons have long favored the local theory of disease, and Cruveilhier's colleagues were no different in that respect. They argued that "the best practical rule to be followed was always to excise [tumors] as early as possible." In other words, they argued for the philosophy more attuned to their own practice.

The debate continued back and forth much in the same way throughout the 1800s. The Pathological Society of London[21] brought greater awareness to the issue when it sponsored a debate in 1874 on cancer as being local versus constitutional, highlighting just how important this topic was for the future of medicine. Nothing conclusive came of this London debate—for better or worse, it ended in stalemate—in large part because the appealingly simple local theory was still favored by many, especially surgeons. In 1879, R. Mitchell[22] reflected on the local theory when he said that "every specific disease depends on one single and indivisible cause for its origin and existence, and not on a combination of causes." The biggest offenders, or at least the most commonly accused, included things like betel nuts, chimney soot, and hot clay pipes. Each was assumed to cause a different type of cancer—oral, scrotal, lip—and each was accepted by surgeons with little resistance.* The aforementioned Bulkley[11,23] ably characterized his contemporaries' narrow-minded focus on single causes of cancer when he said, "The search has been persistently made for some extraneous cause, such as parasitism, (and 'local injury and irritation') but in vain."

Given the popularity of surgery in the contemporary medical establishment, it's unlikely that the local theory could have been overcome. Surgery was unlikely to suddenly disappear or yield to theories of nutritional control.

---

* Incidentally, evidence today shows that single carcinogenic agents at typical levels of exposure are rarely, if ever, enough to increase cancer risk; although early researchers such as Mitchell couldn't have known back then, there's no excuse for the many professionals who remain ignorant today about the questionable evidence supporting a causal role for single cancer-causing chemicals.

Nevertheless, it's possible that the constitutional theory of disease causation might have eventually triumphed, given a little more attention and resources, thus changing the course of history. But it was not to be. Instead of a gradual shift toward the constitutional theory, at the end of the century the debate swung strongly and decisively toward the local theory. This was not because the constitutional theory was proven incorrect, or because surgery had particular excellence, but as a result of two emerging technologies: radiation and chemotherapy. Proponents of the constitutional theory were no longer outnumbered by surgeons alone, but also by a new class of radiotherapists and chemotherapists. By targeting disease at a very precise, local level, these technologies lent themselves to the very same style of treatment as surgery, which left those grappling with the complex metabolism of cancer causation as an even tinier minority.

Following the rise of chemotherapy and radiation, the constitutional theory was progressively delegitimized. The local camp had won, and the human impact of its dominance over the field ever since cannot be overstated. Easy as it may be to get caught up in the more abstract and theoretical levels of this debate, or to philosophize about the appeal of simplicity versus complexity, we must never forget the human element beneath it all. Most importantly, there are the uncountable lives lost as a result of ineffective protocols for cancer prevention and treatment. Anyone who has ever dealt with cancer, as a patient, doctor, or loved one, has been affected by the "progress" made during the early twentieth century. But there are also the many professionals, then as now, who were not only ignored but also punished for their views. Bulkley was expelled from his professional society, the American Association for Cancer Research,[24] at the age of eighty-three for criticizing surgery. And I've already discussed Hoffman's erasure from history, despite his pioneering work and role in the establishment of the ACS.

I also believe that arrogance has had a profound impact on this debate, speeding the dominance of surgery, radiation, and chemotherapy. The belief that vastly complicated diseases can be cured by very simple solutions is at best naïve, but more often simply arrogant. This attitude has continued until relatively recent times, as discussed by celebrated cancer researcher Joan Austoker[25] in reference to breast cancer surgery. Michael Shimkin, perhaps the most influential spokesman in the field of cancer for half a century, perpetuated this belief again in 1957.[26] Also arrogant is the cursory dismissal of alternative views. Did early scientists who were concerned with the complexities of nutritional causation really have nothing to offer? Supporters of the local theory often argued that the constitutional theory was not sufficiently focused and was therefore not even scientific. Such an attitude, in suggesting that there is only one worthy approach to science, is both closed-minded and arrogant. The remarks of W. S. Bainbridge, professor of surgery at the New York Polyclinic Medical School and Hospital, in his 1914 book *The Cancer Problem*,[27] illustrate this arrogance better than most: "that surgical technic [*sic*] has (now) developed to *such a degree of perfection* as to be able [for] one to say with assurance that it is possible to effect a cure of the disease by means of surgical intervention" (emphasis added). (We'll see shortly just how "perfect" that intervention was.) Bainbridge goes on to denigrate skeptics as "the ignorant and . . . timid who fear the knife."

Okay, I admit, this one surpasses arrogance. It is a blatant fallacy—an ad hominem attack focused on the critics of the local theory, rather than their critiques—and nothing short of an assault on logic.

DOMINANT TREATMENT PROTOCOLS

Despite the triumph of the local theory and the celebration surrounding its preferred treatment preferences, the evidence in the early 1900s supporting surgery, radiation, and chemotherapy was not impressive.

Radiotherapy, a treatment method that doses affected areas (e.g., tumors) with high levels of focused radiation in an effort to kill cancer cells, was introduced near the start of the 1900s.[28] It drew considerable interest during the next quarter century, but this interest was not supported by strong evidence. In the largest study of its kind, surgeon Charles L. Gibson[29] reviewed 573 cases of varied cancers for the years 1913 to 1925 at the New York Hospital. He concluded: "Our personal impression is that *no real improvement has been attained* by radiotherapy" (emphasis added).

Despite that conclusion, unwarranted hope for radiotherapy continued to swell. As indicated by the minutes of the ACS national council meeting,[28] the group found it necessary to restrain public optimism in 1914[30] and 1921.[31] In

1925, the managing director of the ACS, George Soper, spoke candidly about the failure of radiation therapy in England.[32] That same year, a series of reports by Hoffman[33] and others[34,35] indicated that excessive radiation exposure was related to *increased* cancer risk and other serious injuries. By 1928,[36] however, the ACS was no longer trying to restrain public confidence in radiation; in fact, they issued a memorandum to ease public fears, so that the disciples of radiotherapy could get on with developing a better product.

By the 1930s, the best that could be said for radiotherapy was the following:

- selective radiotherapy action (i.e., targeted radiation) on cancer cells grown in culture in the laboratory produced inhibited cell growth;
- radiation was simultaneously carcinogenic (promoted cancer by causing mutations) and carcinostatic (restricted cancer by destroying cells, but only if the radiation beam could be focused narrowly enough); and
- useful information on radiotherapy's effectiveness eventually might be found, but only if careful studies in radiobiology were organized.[28]

Contemporary evidence in favor of radiotherapy ranged from unimpressive to nonexistent. Studies that compared the survival rates of patients undergoing radiotherapy as opposed to surgery[29] were perhaps the most impressive. But the data from such studies need to be taken with a handful of salt, for they were fraught with major analytical flaws that I will discuss shortly.

Meanwhile, in the emerging field of chemotherapy—a treatment method that mostly uses highly toxic chemicals in an effort to kill cancer cells*— favorable evidence was virtually nonexistent.[37,38] In fact, chemotherapy was indiscernible from a long line of snake oils used by charlatans, quacks, and well-meaning but misguided physicians of the period. Tellingly, as the concept of chemotherapy became more popular at the turn of the century, it

---

* If that sounds familiar, good; the premise underlying both radiotherapy and chemotherapy is the same: cancer cannot be reversed, only killed.

became more necessary to establish a legal distinction between quack remedies and the remedies of established practitioners.[28] On its face, this sounds
like a good thing. Only a fool would argue against efforts to crack down on
quackery in medicine, right? So you would think. But we should at least
scrutinize the threshold for quackery set by our "established practitioners,"
and see what kind of solutions they proposed.

What we find when we do so is not impressive. In 1926, the ACS organized a landmark conference at Lake Mohonk, New York, to assess the evidence in favor of chemotherapy. According to Francis Carter Wood,[37,38] then
vice president of the ACS and professor of clinical pathology at Columbia University, the best available chemotherapy treatment exhibited there
was the Blair Bell method of intravenously injecting colloidal lead (upward
of 600 mg in one course of treatment). Many other chemicals were also
considered, both during earlier and later years (e.g., selenium in 1912[39] and
1913,[28,40] metabolic inhibitors of respiration, and vital dyes—colorants that
can stain living cells without destroying them).[24,28,41] And what did all these
chemical agents have in common? *No convincing evidence of human efficacy.*

The line between "legitimate" chemotherapy practices based on "scientific principles" and the unscientific products peddled by quacks was apparently very thin. And who were the authorities determining the placement
of that line? Who, for example, sanctioned *intravenously injecting lead* as a
therapy?[37,38] All too clear is that the determination to find a specific cancer antidote was so strong that the ACS was willing to organize trials for
dangerous chemicals.[37,38] During these years, it seems that legitimacy, along
with any respectable standard of evidence, depended most on whose snake
the oil was being extracted from. In short, no reasonable person could have
claimed sufficient evidence for the young and seemingly improvised field of
chemotherapy.*

Last, although contemporary evidence supporting surgery was widely
celebrated, it was no less flawed than the evidence supporting radiation and
chemotherapy.[23,29,37,43] Flaws in the evidence supporting surgery included:

---

* On a more comforting note, this era was not entirely wasted. Anxious to develop chemicals, and especially hormones[42] to treat cancer, there was an increased interest in theoretical
cancer-biology research.

- Failure to statistically control for earlier diagnoses (an early diagnosis, which allows surgeons to go to work earlier, does not establish that surgery is a better cure, and it says nothing about long-term survival, but it does increase the odds of reaching the three-year or five-year benchmark of "survival").
- Giving equal weight to relatively nonfatal cancers and fatal cancers.
- Determining survival rates by comparing cohorts with more operable cases against cohorts with fewer operable cases.
- Categorizing recurrences as "new" cancers, so as to not report the previous surgery as a failure.[23,25,43]
- Reluctance on surgeons' part to count remissions in nonsurgery cases.[23,44]

Despite these serious flaws in the data, there were many who touted the success of surgery. One of the fiercest champions of surgery was Howard Lilienthal, professor of clinical surgery at Cornell.[45] At the 1926 Lake Mohonk ACS conference, he suggested that the most favorable reports on surgery were those of the aforementioned Gibson,[29] surgeon Alexis V. Moschcowitz,[43] and M. Greenwood.[37] But these sources, especially the first two, were distorted by Lilienthal.

When I compared Lilienthal's conference account[45] of Gibson's study with Gibson's own account,[29] I found only blatant misrepresentation. Gibson was a surgeon at the Cornell Division of the New York Hospital, and his report documented the follow-up histories of 573 cases of varied cancers between 1913 and 1925. Here's what he had to say about surgery and the evidence so many used to support it: "We have been living in *a fool's paradise of fallacious statistics* . . . and all the older figures should be ruthlessly junked and so-called radical operations should only be performed after the most painstaking search for metastases is exhausted" (emphasis added).[29] Lilienthal completely ignored this account and perverted Gibson's data to reach a much different conclusion: "The chances, with surgery, of remaining alive for a given period are double those without its aid in the same length of time." He went on to say that "many of the cases reported are fine examples of operative skill and surgical judgement with results brilliant in the extreme." Results *brilliant in the extreme*? What a far cry from Gibson's own account:

"No sadder report of the disheartening status of cancer surgery has come to our attention."

I have the luxury of hindsight, and of being able to highlight these reports' differences through side-by-side excerpts, as if in dialogue. Sadly, Gibson was unable to defend his report's findings in the same way, because he wasn't even invited to the 1926 ACS conference. Despite being the architect and author of the most comprehensive study of its kind, he was left at home. Shamefully, so were the devastating results of his study. And clearly Gibson's exclusion from the conference was not the result of an innocent oversight, considering that Lilienthal was obviously aware of his work and willing to "analyze" (misconstrue) it in his absence.

Likewise, the actual results of Moschcowitz et al.'s research[43] at Mt. Sinai Hospital in New York (also celebrated at the conference) were mysteriously omitted from Lilienthal's paper, and it's not hard to see Lilienthal's motivations. Lilienthal began by praising the (subsequently recognized as macabre) Halstead mastectomy and concluded by stating that "the modern operation is usually successful in eradicating the local process, as is evidenced by the very large number of cases dying from distant metastases, without even a suspicion of a recurrence." But his claim that metastases were not even suspected of being recurrences directly contradicts Moschcowitz, who made a point of saying that it wasn't possible to distinguish for sure between recurrences and metastases. Moschcowitz also cautioned that survival rates "are not as favorable as one might be led to believe from a cursory examination of the literature."

Meanwhile, arguments that opposed surgery during this time also included those* of Robert Bell,[46] J. Shaw,[47] and Bulkley;[23] Austoker's review notes additional dissent.[25] Taking those critiques into account, as well as the contemporary and more recent analytic reviews of the practice, the flawed data that supported surgery, and the intense emotionalism and bias surrounding the entire issue,[25,48,49] it's clear that surgery's early twentieth-century

---

* Dr. Bell rejected surgery after many years of practice, and when attempting to inform his colleagues of his disenchantment with it, encountered great hostility and professional ostracism. After considerable frustration, he wrote a book to tell his story, depositing copies in a few key libraries. Upon discovering his book, I had to separate uncut pages in two places; obviously I was the first reader of his book in the Bodleian Library at Oxford in eighty years!

dominance (alongside radiotherapy and chemotherapy) was not won or justified by merit alone.

EVIDENCE FROM THE SAME PERIOD SUPPORTING NUTRITION

Treatment of cancer is more urgent and personal than prevention of cancer. Thus, treatment tends to attract a focused approach like those offered by surgery, chemotherapy, and radiotherapy, where cancer is approached as a local disease to be treated locally. Nutrition did not offer this possibility during the late 1800s (and neither does it now!), partly because many types of nutrients, which might hypothetically focus their effects, had not yet been discovered. Thus, with the growing philosophical adoption of the local theory, combined with the urgency of treatment, nutrition's association with cancer was not considered a possibility for cancer treatment. Nutrition was a constitutional or lifestyle effect that, at best, might only help prevent cancer.

Nutrition's potential effect on cancer prevention, however, eventually led to several types of human studies: studies that compared the cancer mortality rates of populations with nutrient patterns and gradations of dietary practice; time-trend comparisons of mortality rates given the availability of certain foods; studies that observed a correlation among migration, food-consumption trends, and cancer risk (i.e., how cancer risk rose or fell as individuals or groups moved and adopted new diets); and at least one very large case-control study (in Hoffman's case). Early experimental animal studies (1913–1914)[50,51] also showed that lower calorie consumption significantly reduced growth of transplanted tumor tissue.

The most convincing evidence of cancer's association with lifestyle and environment was illustrated by the effects of migration on cancer risk. As mentioned in chapter two, this was a favorite form of evidence for Hoffman,[52] Williams,[15] Russell,[8] and many others. The most common hypothesis was that "excessive" nutrition was responsible for cancer. How else could they explain that cancer rates were highest among the most "robust" and seemingly healthy members of the population? In 1908, Williams[15] proposed that excessive nutrition sparked tumor growth at the cellular level, until eventually that tumor exhibited growth independence or "proliferative power." On the effects of external versus internal factors in tumor development, he said, "It is probable that in the past, the value of extrinsic factors, as formative stimuli, have been underrated; it, nevertheless, seems probable, from the whole course of cancer growth, that, in tumor formation, as in normal growth, intrinsic factors usually predominate." Here, "intrinsic factors" refers to complex functions of metabolism; in other words, a constitutional origin of disease.

None of this evidence in support of nutrition was esoteric. It was well known throughout the period, especially among the most powerful leaders in cancer research and education societies. Hoffman could not have been clearer in his 1913 "Menace of Cancer" speech, which led to the founding of the ACS. He made ten recommendations for the new society, most of them encouraging improved statistical procedures and data for recording cancer prevalence among different populations. But he also made two very specific recommendations on determining the causes of cancer: that "incidences of occupational hazards with respect to cancer be exactly determined" and that "nutritional influences on the induction of cancer be analyzed." In the history of the society written by E. H. Rigney,[53] Hoffman specifically said, "Since an erroneous diet is a probable causative factor in cancer occurrence, the nutrition of cancerous patients should be investigated in conformity with . . . strictly scientific and conclusive methods." Although the new society embraced Hoffman's recommendation on the development of statistical surveys, they ignored his recommendations to study nutritional and environmental factors. And this early neglect set a pattern that has dominated the ACS ever since.

Nutritional theories were also well known in Britain. A major study on diet and cancer among religious orders,[37] conducted by the British Empire Cancer Campaign (BECC), acknowledged in 1926 that "certain English medical men, whose names deservedly carry great weight," took nutrition seriously and, furthermore, that "a bibliography on the subject of diet and cancer would extend to many hundred titles."

Unfortunately, to return to the central point of interest, everything changed toward the end of the nineteenth century when the local theory of cancer causation became dominant. Its dominance is clearly reflected in the medical practice of that time and in the medical practice since. The dominance of surgery, chemotherapy, and radiotherapy, in the *absence* of convincing evidence, testifies to the power of dogma; the disregard for other protocols, in the *presence* of evidence, testifies to a longstanding tendency toward repressing controversial views. These tendencies became even more predominant in the early twentieth century with the rise of several cancer institutions.

THE RISE OF INSTITUTIONS

We have seen so far how the local theory of cancer causation triumphed over the constitutional theory around the turn of the twentieth century, and how that affected our approaches to both treatment and the irresponsible misrepresentation of data. Why this battle and so many of its participants have been deleted from the history of cancer research, and why the same questionable theory and practices regarding cancer causation and treatment persist today, can be explained by the formation of a few powerful cancer institutions in the early 1900s: the Imperial Cancer Research Fund (ICRF), the American Association for Cancer Research (AACR), the ACS introduced in chapter two, and the BECC. The power of these four institutions was, and remains, inescapable. Nearly all professional activities concerning cancer research have been developed, funded, and controlled by these institutions, in addition to one more: the US government's all-powerful, taxpayer-funded National Cancer Institute (NCI) of the National Institutes of Health (NIH), which was founded by leaders of the ACS and the AACR.

Obvious though it may be, it's important to remember that institutions begin as nothing more than groups of like-minded people, and that groups of like-minded people tend to become increasingly like-minded as time passes. This is a matter of human nature: as with any group of humans seeking harmony and stability, professional institutions tend to encourage conformity far more than outstanding individual opinion. Even among groups of self-identified outsiders (I'm thinking here of various countercultural movements), the process of grouping eventually bears conformity. When paired with tremendous power, such conformity becomes a dangerous force, limiting public will and tending toward institutional self-preservation and stagnation. This is true even when the vast majority of individuals within an institution have nothing but the best intentions.

Debates among independent and freethinking individuals—say, for example, nineteenth-century debates about the constitutional versus local theories of cancer causation—may be fiery and controversial, but they are at least more permissive of minority opinions than the same debates within an institution whose position already has been established. Minority opinions are less likely to be expressed, for fear of reprisal—no one wants to be shunned or exiled from their professional society—and so the character of the debates themselves shifts, too. Always one eye is fixed on the party line; independent individuals are downgraded and bunched into homogeneous hives, and freethinking is subsumed by groupthink (which I describe further in chapter five).

Bleak as this may sound, the histories of our most celebrated cancer societies illustrate this pattern all too well. Both in Great Britain and the United States, these organizations were founded and controlled by a small and exclusive group of medical authorities, whose biases uniformly favored the local theory of disease causation and their own treatment protocols. Unsurprisingly, and without exception, none of them gave credence to the recommendations for research on nutrition made by Williams in 1908[15] and Hoffman in 1913.[52] They neglected those recommendations, I'd suggest, not as a matter of conspiracy, but due to a combination of more mundane human defects like stubbornness, bias, and conformity. By these forces, both conscious and subconscious, they settled on recommendations more to their liking. Also, they were clearly influenced by the for-profit sector, which embraced the local theory of disease because it supported the marketing of products.

Why did no institutions arise to support the constitutional theory of cancer causation? Despite the evidence in nutrition's favor, the emerging fields of chemotherapy and radiotherapy had a greater potential for profit, because they lent themselves to the continued and simultaneous discovery of identifiable cancer-fighting products. Further, since the development of new chemical agents and cancer-fighting technology was amenable to intellectual property protection needed for the marketplace, funding was far easier to obtain. Last, the public had no reason to distrust the four primary cancer societies. Though public skepticism toward the health care system is not uncommon today, projecting this recent fashion onto attitudes of the past century would be a mistake. We were younger then, more trustful of institutions, and not yet the mass victims of chronic disease. As a result, there was virtually nothing to counterbalance the institutions' impact on our society's health, and no one to question their inordinate influence.

EXAMPLES OF INSTITUTIONAL BIASES

Few individuals exerted a greater influence over British cancer research efforts than Ernest Bashford, the ICRF's first research director and the man responsible for outlining the organization's original research plan. He was also deeply predisposed toward the local theory of cancer causation. In 1914,[54] he denied Hoffman's proposition that cancer rates were increasing in the Western world.[52] He referred to a 1905 ICRF report on cancer statistics, written by himself and J. A. Murray, concluding (as I mentioned in chapter two) that statistics on cancer rates in Ireland were less accurate than those from England, and that statistics from poorer countries on the periphery of the British Empire were even less reliable. Based on this interpretation of the statistics, Bashford claimed, the nutritional hypothesis, which largely depends on statistical analyses of population characteristics, was seriously flawed, and England had nothing to worry about. Unfortunately for Bashford and the English nation, this was pure speculation.

The report went further still: "As was to be expected from the facts already made known [from the first ICRF report] . . . diet exerts no primary influence on the occurrence of cancer in various races of mankind." Besides a purely speculative dismissal of data accuracy based on the national origins of that data, how did Bashford and the ICRF justify their disregard for large-scale statistical studies linking nutrition to cancer?

Bashford and Murray's ulterior motives are revealed elsewhere in the report. They claim that "it has been proved that cancer is only experimentally transmissible by actual transplantation of tissues," and further, "it is useless to attempt to establish by statistical means such as a cancer census a relationship between sporadic cases of cancer." Now, if this sounds confusing to you, don't worry—it should! After all, what do statistical efforts to trace cancer rates have to do with tumor implantation studies? There's no obvious conflict between these two points; why should they be mutually exclusive, or even compete at all?

Why, then, did Bashford and Murray even make a point of discussing tumor transplant studies in this report? When I discovered that ICRF's research efforts at the time were disproportionately focused on tumor transplantation studies, and that Bashford's own personal research experience was concerned with this very topic,[24] everything else slid into place. Bashford and Murray's neglect for statistical studies had less to do with the studies themselves and more to do with their own preestablished research interests, and the interests of their institution. To claim that data from Ireland and less-developed parts of the world are somehow tainted is to find an easy way out of taking those findings seriously, or of having to make a meaningful connection between transplantation studies and statistical analyses.

Regardless of where this bias originated, their insistence on singing the praises of tumor transplant studies, in a seemingly unrelated report on cancer statistics, sounds an awful lot like upper management toeing the company line. It suggests to me that Bashford and Murray weren't all that interested in an honest assessment of nutrition, or in fact any other perspective that didn't fit neatly into the ICRF's existing research agenda.

Such bias continued to dominate cancer research in Great Britain throughout World War I. There was, however, a concern among medical professionals that the ICRF was too focused on laboratory research and wasn't funding enough clinical research.[55] To meet this need, another group of doctors organized the BECC. In the first year after its formation in 1923, there was quite a bit of political maneuvering behind the scenes. The secretary of the British Medical Research Council (MRC), Walter Morley Fletcher, demanded control of the newly formed BECC, including its propaganda and publicity effort, to effectively steer how the public would perceive cancer and its treatment.[55] With help from the Board of Trade, he achieved this control within the year. This effectively gave him the power to funnel BECC funds directly into those areas of cancer research favored by the MRC, and especially toward his own radiobiological investigations.[55]

Considering its preoccupation with MRC-mandated research topics, it's unsurprising that the BECC published almost nothing about nutrition, whether supporting its involvement in cancer or rejecting it. Still, two exceptions stand out: "The Truth About Cancer" in 1930,[56] and a report written four years later by surgeon John Percy Lockhart-Mummery.[57] The second of these reports[58] took an especially aggressive stance against nutrition research: "Various suggestions have been put forward that the incidence of cancer is related to certain foods, or absence of foods, but there is no evidence whatever to support such an idea, and a very great deal of evidence to refute it." I find this quote interesting, given that the BECC had ignored nutrition for nearly all of its early history. Why did they suddenly feel the need to call out nutrition? Were they threatened by the increasing evidence in favor of a nutritional hypothesis? I can only speculate, but the Lockhart-Mummery report does seem to mark a change in strategy. After ignoring nutrition for some time, the BECC seemed here to move toward a more proactive smear campaign.

Other attempts to undermine the evidence supporting nutrition were generally clumsy and dishonest. In one instance, the BECC claimed that "experimental investigations in animals to test these theories have so far been *entirely* negative"; later, the report casts doubt on the "*supposed* unequal geographical distribution of cancer" (both emphases added). This uncompromising refusal to consider the nutritional hypothesis echoes the earlier claims made in 1930's "The Truth About Cancer": "There is no shred of reliable evidence that consumption of or abstinence from any particular article of diet leads to the occurrence of cancer, and that *definite* evidence exists that there is no difference in the liability to cancer of strictly vegetarian communities" (emphasis added).[56] Not only are most of these claims patently false, they also demonstrate the systemic closed-mindedness and intolerance that Hoffman lamented in *Cancer and Diet*.[10]

These bold conclusions rely on a 1926 study by Copeman and Greenwood.[37] Sponsored by the BECC itself, the study claimed to have found no difference in cancer rates among selected religious orders consuming a vegetarian diet. Naturally, I took considerable interest in this study. What I found was not convincing evidence against nutrition, but rather one of the most wickedly misinterpreted studies I've ever read (although I know of some good present-day competitors). Death certificate data showing lower cancer rates among religious houses adhering to a vegetarian diet were deformed in all manner of ways:

- The authors artificially increased apparent cancer rates in vegetarian houses by rediagnosing death certificates (i.e., renaming the cause of death) and by counting "probable" cases, but made no such adjustments when figuring cancer death rates among the general population.
- When they found cancer incidence rates of only 20 to 40 percent of the expected rate among a large cohort of Continental European houses practicing vegetarianism, they discarded the data.
- They further obfuscated the data by using irrelevant statistical analogies and also alleged a greater practice of vegetarianism than really existed.
- Corresponding to their interest in degrading claims favoring a vegetarian practice, they suggested a conclusion based on Hoffman's study of Indigenous peoples in North America[59] that was the complete opposite of what Hoffman himself had concluded.

Even with all that, the data in Copeman and Greenwood's study showed that the religious houses most strictly observing vegetarianism had the fewest cases of cancer, categorized as having "exceedingly rare" occurrences or none.

Apparently, this escaped the authors' notice. They conclude: "A perusal of our report will convince most impartial persons that no scientific value whatever attaches to assertions, supported merely by the vague pseudo-statistical evidence which is customarily cited, respecting the roles of certain articles of common consumption in the genesis of cancer."

* * *

It would be difficult to discuss these institutions and their biases without including a word on some of their most prominent leaders, like Charles

Childe,[60] who was president of the British Medical Association when the BECC was founded. In 1923 he claimed that "the most important fact we know about [cancer] is that in its beginnings it is local and that its course is a centrifugal spread from its local point of origin." Sounds familiar, right? This is the local theory of disease, cemented as "truth" by institutional authority. As for the concept of centrifugal spread—the idea that diseases spread from a single, central point of origin (local disease origin)—Childe inherited this from the earlier observations of W. Sampson Handley,[61] a very influential surgeon at the Middlesex Hospital cancer ward, which was founded all the way back in 1792.[62] Handley's theory of centrifugal spread is an exceedingly rudimentary explanation for an exceedingly complex problem. Nevertheless, it was very influential. According to Austoker's review,[25] it had provided the supposedly scientific basis for William Halstead's "macabre" radical mastectomy, introduced at the end of the nineteenth century.[63]

Besides developing the theory of centrifugal spread, Handley was also vocally opposed to large-scale statistical studies, or those that can identify the spread of risk factors across many people at the same time—the opposite of the local-origin theory of disease. In 1931,[64] he disputed such studies as well as any nutritional hypotheses that they might have suggested. His adherence to the local theory of cancer causation is reflected in his preference for narrowly focused research methods. Rather than statistical studies, Handley favored "the patient study of *individual* cases of the disease" (emphasis added). He additionally referred to the work of Charles Moore, surgeon at the Middlesex Hospital. According to Handley, Moore proved the local theory of causation "in 1867. . . [when he] showed that recurrence after operation is due, not to an organic or constitutional taint, but to incomplete removal of the primary growth and its surrounding satellite nodules." It's easy to see how this theory, and its emphasis on early and complete removal of the so-called primary growths, eventually inspired Halstead's use of radical mastectomy.

Handley claimed further success on behalf of the local theory by celebrating the success of "local treatment by radium." On that point, it bears repeating that in 1925 Hoffman[33] and others[34,35] showed that radiation therapy *increased* cancer risk, and that even Handley's American counterparts at the ACS had actively tried to *restrain* public optimism for this practice in the preceding decades.[30] But like so many before and after him, Handley was unperturbed by these contradictions. In fact, he continued to speak out in favor of the local theory in his 1955 book *The Genesis and Prevention of Cancer*.[65] In that book, he also revealed a startling fondness for authoritarian information control and "direct public propaganda" disseminated by institutions like the BECC. Although he hedged somewhat by labeling this propaganda "of secondary importance" to the institution's mission, compared to the goal of promoting surgery, he was not shy in discussing its potential. (Has the term "spin doctor" ever been more apt?)

The fate of the nutrition–cancer hypothesis in Britain was sealed by 1936, when the Health Education and Research Council published its survey on cancer research.[66] Its author, Maurice Beddow Bayly, flippantly dismissed nutrition: "This need not detain us long, for the reason that throughout the entire history of investigations carried out under the two great research funds the writer has failed to discover anything whatsoever that might be dignified by the term 'scientific'"—when, as we have seen, research spanning decades, including experimental animal studies, human population studies, and empirical accounts, showed a connection to nutrition.

I'm reminded here, once again, of both the arrogance of science's gatekeepers in selectively disregarding certain types of research, and of the power of institutional definition. By the latter I mean these organizations' unopposed ability to define one thing as scientific and another as unscientific, merely because it suits their interests. The organizations described above limited "science" to research that adhered to the local theory, a stance that the cancer establishment has carried forth to the present. This institutional definition is all about maintaining power structures, so that influential doctors like Bayly can maintain complete control. Thus, the absence of nutrition from the "great research funds" of Britain is neither a surprise nor an argument against nutrition; it is merely the policy of those institutions and further proof of their biases.

Last, even though the evidence wasn't originating from the BECC or the ICRF, evidence for a nutritional association *did* exist. Bayly obviously felt the need to address some of this evidence, particularly the increasing number of animal studies showing the effect of diet on tumor development. But again, he dismissed these findings, asserting that animal studies "can produce no results of any value, and the experiments would be ludicrous if it were not for . . . the tragic delay in the progress of scientific knowledge . . . it is surely unnecessary to comment upon the scientific valuelessness of such inanities." Surely unnecessary to comment? And yet he couldn't restrain his own comment, blurting the words "ludicrous" and "inanities" like an impulsive ventriloquist torn between science and the script that ruled him.

* * *

In the United States, the AACR and the ACS were just as beholden as British organizations to the dogmatic research biases of their founding fathers: both denied the role of nutrition in cancer development. This dogma permeated all levels of research funding, choice of experimental methods, and publication. It also carried over to the founding of the NCI as a government agency in 1937. The NCI went on to become the most dominant cancer research agency in the world, a position it maintains today.

The professional backgrounds of the AACR's early leaders illustrate this point well. Of the eleven charter members in 1907, nine were either surgeons or pathologists. None had any background whatsoever in nutrition. Much like the ICRF, the AACR's founders were enamored with the recent wave of tumor transplant studies. In particular, they were very excited about the work of two groups of researchers, one in England and one in the US.[24] The hope at the time was that, by studying tumor transplants, researchers might discover some kind of cancer immunity.

I can understand the appeal of these early studies. But that doesn't justify the exclusion of research on nutritional effects, particularly when other avenues of research didn't face nearly as many obstacles. In fact, the AACR focused great attention on surgery, X-radiation, radium, and "caustic [lye-based] pastes," and their hunt for biological materials with carcinostatic (cancer-halting) potential gave great momentum to the rising field of chemotherapy, which was still struggling to find its feet.[24] Notably, this focus on carcinostatics may have stemmed from G. H. A. Clowes (one of the two non-surgeon, non-pathologist charter members of the AACR), who argued that cancer was caused by a virus. Clowes's example demonstrates just how important representation in these research organizations can be: it's quite likely that Clowes's inclusion among the charter members was directly responsible for the ramped-up search for immunization procedures that might have the potential to inhibit cancer growth.[67] Unfortunately, nutrition had no such advocate.

But the AACR's contempt for nutrition was not only obvious by its negligence. They also had a very low tolerance for dissent. Bulkley,[24] the chief organizer and first director of the New York Skin and Cancer Hospital, learned this the hard way when, despite his distinguished background and faultless reputation, the AACR decided to excommunicate him for merely suggesting that there was a nonsurgical way to treat cancer.[25] Let's be perfectly clear: there was nothing especially showy or incendiary about Bulkley's small and isolated revolt, if it can even be called a revolt. He simply spoke out about the shortcomings of surgery, particularly breast surgery,[25] in a time when many of his colleagues believed surgery was God's perfect procedure. According to Hoffman,[10] Bulkley also questioned why nutrition "had never yet been given a fair and fully intelligent trial." Two years later, he restated this point with greater conviction and more convincing evidence. Citing the findings of more than thirty-five cancer surgeons, he concluded that no more than one in ten cancer patients could expect a cure from surgery.[23]

I'm not sure whether the AACR was more incensed by Bulkley's advocacy of nutrition or by the evidence he provided against surgery. I suspect it was a combination. And at the end of the day, it doesn't really matter. Both were considered cardinal sins.

Despite Hoffman's early involvement and later research contributions,[24,52,68] introduced in chapter two, the ACS was no more tolerant of the nutritional hypothesis than the AACR. Hoffman's continued work in and around the ACS, despite never being truly welcome, says less about the society's impartiality than it does about his own impressive stature. There was surely a time when the society would have been happy to get rid of him. But by the time he delivered that de facto inaugural speech, he had already established a reputation as the preeminent statistician in the country.

Besides, his persistence did not guarantee the support and respect of the ACS's leading authorities. While not entirely silenced, his recommendations were only ever taken selectively and his impact only ever rewarded minimally. He was kept at arm's length and never given due credit. For example, when he was awarded the ACS's seventh annual Clement Cleveland Medal, there was no mention of his contributions and recommendations on nutrition. Unfortunately, he was unable to accept the award in person, due to failing health.

Among the six pre-Hoffman recipients of the ACS Medal, four were media and fundraising individuals and organizations, and two were scientists.[24,53] James Ewing was one of those scientists. As well as being a charter member of the society in 1913 and a professor of pathology at Cornell Medical School, Ewing was a prominent charter member of the AACR and an original member of the National Cancer Advisory Council (NCAC) of the NCI in 1937. In other words, there were very few scientists in cancer circles, if any, whose influence could have surpassed Ewing's in the first forty years of the twentieth century;[24,53] given that, it's no surprise that he would have been awarded the Cleveland Medal before Hoffman. But I think it also speaks to the priorities of the ACS. At the symposium dedicated to Ewing,[69] Welch emphasized that Ewing's recognition was "abundantly justified by the strikingly improved results of treatment by *radical surgery* or by *radiotherapy*" (emphasis added).[70]

The other pre-Hoffman scientist recipient of the award was Frances Carter Wood, director of the Institute of Cancer Research at Columbia University. Like Ewing, he also represented ACS on the NCAC and his research interests aligned with mainstream treatment, especially the Blair Bell colloidal-lead method. Again, it's no surprise that Wood, Ewing, and big donors would have received the Cleveland Award before Hoffman. The pattern was set.

In the grand scheme of things, the award itself doesn't matter. It's not my place, a hundred years later, to claim victimization on Hoffman's behalf. However, what is important is what it tells us about these institutions and their biases during this formative period.

Though the ACS didn't have its own formal research program until the 1940s, it did exercise considerable control over discourse in the field of cancer, ensuring a joint stranglehold (along with the AACR) on practically all cancer research until the formation of the NCI. Crucially, it also controlled the flow of information, determining what topics were suitable for debate and under what circumstances. This power is clear in its NCI involvement, its National Cancer Advisory Council, the *Journal of Cancer Research* (now called the *Journal of the National Cancer Institute*),[24,53] and the seminal inaugural Lake Mohonk research conference.[53] It was in journals like these and at conferences like this where the most important debates on cancer took place, and where the very parameters of those debates were established. Of the NCAC's initial seven members, the ACS selected four, plus the chair.

Unsurprisingly, when Ewing and others who later became NCAC members prepared the roster of speakers for the Lake Mohonk conference,[53] they excluded outliers like Hoffman and radiology critic Gibson. Given that the conference was focused heavily on the interpretation of cancer statistics and mortality trends, the exclusion of Hoffman is especially reprehensible. Nearly every one of the thirty-one presenters was either a surgeon, a pathologist, or a specialist in clinical medicine. There were no nutritionists and only one statistician, a virtual unknown. In his talk,[71] Ewing belittled recommendations on diet and cancer as "semi-medical literature," and showed his favoritism for targeted radiation as a means of treatment—a means, I might add, in which he had invested a large chunk of his own professional life.[70]

FORGETFULNESS IS BLISS

When I emerged from this densely wooded history of nutrition and cancer research at Oxford in 1986, it was with a new pair of eyes. Looking back on that history, I'm more impressed than ever by how many lessons it contains on the formation of our most cherished beliefs about nutrition and cancer—many of which persist today—and their suspect origins, too. Some may point out that this history is deeper than what I've covered here, and surely messier. I won't deny this point. (Isn't history always deeper and messier than our narratives can contain?) Neither will I presume to understand every level of irrationality in the cancer research community. Though I've highlighted a few elements—the appeal of overly simplistic explanations, the pervasiveness of professional biases, and the power of institutions—there are other possible reasons why priorities have been low for research on nutrition and cancer. For example, diet has always been closely tied to tradition and class hierarchy. I don't know the exact degree of impact, but it's possible these and other elements also played an important role in the rejection of nutritional hypotheses.

To keep this discussion accessible and reasonably succinct, I had to make choices about which events and reports to include. I could have cited many more authors, medical authorities, and scientists for further emphasis. As much as possible, I based my decisions on which to include on two things: the prominence of the individual writer and my ability to read firsthand accounts. In doing so, I hope to have appropriately represented the field and accurately reflected the authors' views.

However, with these limitations in mind, I noticed certain well-documented patterns emerging:

1. Theory determines practice, and vice versa. The victory of the local theory over the constitutional theory reinforces the victory of surgery, radiotherapy, and chemotherapy over nutrition, and the apparently successful (even if for a short duration) use of local treatments reinforces our belief in the local theory.

2. Practice, in turn, shapes the formation of institutions. If more practitioners had taken the "vegetable diet"[72] of the early 1800s seriously, then perhaps they might have formed a research institution of their own and raised funds for studies.

3. Finally, institutions circle back to shape the discourse, including through national policy, surrounding theory, and practice. Their biases tend toward the theories and practices they know best, the same theories and practices that were their makers, thus perpetuating the vicious cycle. This is most intentional when they protect economically rewarding practices.

Within this schema are a vast number of individuals, many with good intentions. My view on these individuals is simple: their good intentions have been institutionalized. Their valiant efforts have been imprisoned, their philanthropy locked up. They have become stuck in a loop, and so has the society that receives their messaging. Crucially, they have also forgotten their own institutionalization. In the foundational years of these institutions, the constitutional theory and nutrition were ignored, uninvited, disincentivized;

later, they were outright forgotten, even erased from these institutions' histories because they deviated from what had become known as science itself.

Moving forward, we might say that the greatest threats to human health are not the ineffectual strategies and protocols that we call "treatments," costly and damaging though they may be, but rather the far more enveloping practice of forgetfulness. If institutions are harsh in their treatment of nonconformists, it is likely not because the participants in this enterprise (researchers, policy makers, etc.) are evil conspirators, but because they have ignored or forgotten the past. They are out of touch with the relevant and important work that preceded them. This is a problem for all scientists, but it is especially detrimental when it comes to research on biologically complex diseases like cancer: we focus far too much attention on the near future, on framing questions and designing projects, and not nearly enough attention on surveying and integrating past lessons.

During the early part of my career, it was generally accepted that any new research project should be preceded by a review of past literature, generally going back at least a couple of decades. Now, it seems that anything published more than five years ago is considered outdated, even irrelevant. As more and more people have entered research, the pace and amount of publishing has accelerated, and "history" is now squeezed from only a few years prior.

I tried to confront this issue some forty years ago when I was on sabbatical leave at the headquarters of the Federation of American Societies for Experimental Biology and Medicine outside of Washington, DC. While there, I was appointed to a Congressional liaison position responsible for monitoring biomedical research funding in Congress. It was an overwhelming job that involved far more lobbying and politicking than I could put up with. Frankly, I did a rather poor job; it was not a good fit for my persona. In any case, as the first academic to have held that position, I was asked to summarize my thoughts, experiences, and whatever useful guidelines I might have for possible successors. Mindful of the environment I was working in, in which most were focused on the near future, with little regard for lessons from the past, I came up with a somewhat tongue-in-cheek suggestion: that we shut down all new NIH research funding (except for ongoing salaries) for five years and instead devote the time and funding to holding conferences and deliberating on the lessons of the past century. I suggested that we might give the future of biomedical research a new direction by mapping the old routes.

My senior colleagues thought this upstart idea was crazy; everyone knew that the research enterprise, narrow though it was, was moving along *just* right without the need for further deliberation, and that any such discussion would hamper the all-important forward momentum of science (never mind where that force was taking us). In the end, the federation did not want to publish my paper[73] and I relented. Their view was that such a statement would cast too much light on inefficiency within NIH. I agreed that they had a good point. But remember, that was forty years ago! We now have far more scientific information to organize, translate, and put to good use. Most of it will never see the light of day. Most will be forgotten before the ink dries. And so, the wheel of science will continue its spin, not forward on the earth like a tire, but hoisted and fixed to the frame of our institutions, perpetually, redundantly turning.

Research and treatment today must fit within an ever-narrowing scope. I have no doubt that if it were possible to distill the power of nutrition into a single, identifiable agent, like a pill or a procedure, then it would receive much more support and representation. Meanwhile, the old treatment protocols championed by the local theory of disease more than a hundred years ago continue to dominate the field of cancer, despite their ineffectiveness. Indeed, if these had been effective treatment protocols from the beginning—if the results were truly "brilliant in the extreme" as some commentators asserted—then we might have completely avoided the so-called war on cancer introduced in chapter one.

Instead, that war rages on.

Our modern, "advanced" approach to cancer treatment inflicts mind-numbing costs and often-fatal physical trauma. According to 2014 estimates, the average cost of a round of treatment for office-managed chemotherapy is approximately $20,000; for hospital-managed chemotherapy, the price rises to $26,000.[74] Worse still, these costs are rising faster than the average cost of living, so that many individual patients today must make the impossible choice between forgoing treatment and being consumed by medical bills. It's disgusting that so many citizens of such a wealthy country should be financially devastated by the mere effort to stay alive. I'm sure most would agree. And as we've seen, the effectiveness of many of these efforts is highly questionable at best. According to a 2004 joint Australian-American research group that assessed a large body of data concerning twenty-two types of cancer, our "treatment" is no treatment at all. Five-year survival rates for patients using cytotoxic chemotherapy drugs increased by an average of only 2.1 percent[75] compared to nontreatment, a significant portion of which may be attributed to nothing more than the placebo effect. And if that isn't bad enough, a recent report from the European Medicines Agency found that the majority (57 percent) of authorized cancer drugs between 2009 and 2013 came to market *without any evidence* that "they improved the quality or quantity of patients' lives."[76] Yet, many were introduced in the marketplace as "breakthrough therapies." This "quality or quantity" threshold for measuring success is not very specific or rigorous. It doesn't even distinguish between short- versus long-term effects. Yet most drugs released during the surveyed time frame failed to show this benefit. So poisonous are our cancer "medicines" that patients are directed to flush their toilets twice after using them.[77] This is important because the medication stays in your body for about 48 hours after treatment and it can harm healthy people in your home. And if it can harm healthy people, what might this "medication" be doing to the extremely ill patients who receive it?

In short, though many decades have passed, our ability to treat cancer has not improved. We have merely "updated" the ineffective treatments of one hundred years ago, and all because we have continued to misunderstand and ignore nutrition's role in causing and potentially treating this disease.

REMEMBERING THE ALTERNATIVE

The whole food, plant-based (WFPB) diet and its supporting research are controversial because they challenge the prevailing cultural narrative that diet and disease are only partially and narrowly related. In the last two chapters we have discussed this in the context of cancer, but the predominance of this cultural narrative is more or less apparent for all diseases. My preference for discussing cancer is based on my own expertise in the area and the rich history that I uncovered in Oxford during the mid-'80s. But make no mistake: the same broad lessons apply to other fields of disease as well.

What I hope to have shown here is that this narrative is a relatively recent phenomenon, in the grand scheme of things. There exists no indisputable mandate to justify our exclusive belief in local causes and local treatments. The evidence in the early twentieth century did not warrant adopting an exclusive belief in local causes and local treatments, and neither does the evidence today. Why should we persist in that exclusive belief, given the costs? Has the time not finally come to give something else a try, as William Lambe proposed two hundred years ago?

The WFPB diet is controversial because it resurrects that old debate about local versus constitutional disease. The status quo today proclaims that this debate has already been put to bed, but the research supporting the WFPB diet suggests otherwise. By establishing the connection between nutrition and disease, it resurrects an old source of controversy—one that the status quo would much rather continue forgetting.

But it's not only the broken disease-care system that the WFPB diet challenges. As I will discuss in Part II, it also challenges our conventional understanding of "good" nutrition, especially orthodox attitudes toward animal protein.

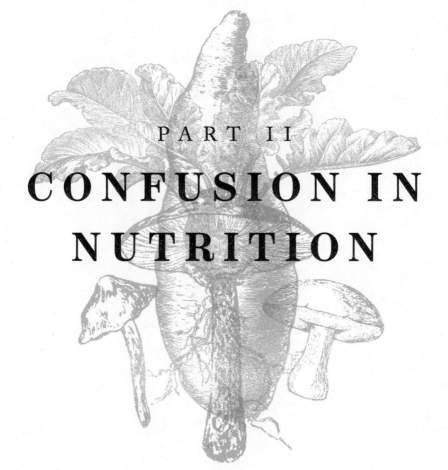

PART II

CONFUSION IN NUTRITION

CHAPTER FOUR

THE STATE OF
NUTRITION

I had nothing to offer anybody except my own confusion.
—Jack Kerouac

I wish the problems facing us were simpler, and that three chapters were enough. I wish we could simply say: *Great! Nutrition has a powerful role to play in the formation of disease and the promotion of health. Now let's* do *it.* Unfortunately, I cannot. Just as our attitudes toward the association of nutrition with disease (or lack thereof) are wedded to the questionable narratives more than a century old, so too are our attitudes toward the science of nutrition itself. Just as contrary viewpoints are dismissed in the former, so too are they dismissed in the latter. What this means is that even *if* it were universally accepted that nutrition has a powerful role to play in both disease and health, many would remain confused about what optimal nutrition really *looks like.*

Consider your own experience and I am sure you will think of plenty of examples. The divisive, confusing discourse surrounding health and nutrition

83

has become almost unavoidable. Our attitudes toward health and nutrition are critically important in determining the *diets* we prefer, either directly or indirectly, and few could dispute the fractiousness that has come to define modern dieting. Whether you favor a caveman-in-the-twenty-first-century diet; a high-fat, emergency-state diet; a prelapsarian, prefire vegan diet; or perhaps some pick-and-choose combination of these and other popular diets, chances are you've witnessed the stubborn defensiveness and counterattacks that such camps breed. Additionally, numerous ethical, environmental, and religious justifications influence our dietary choices. Much like in our current political landscape, we're at an impasse, and getting past that impasse requires a seismic shift in the way we consider not only diet, but also the underlying attitudes we have toward health and nutrition.

I have been caught in the crossfire of diet debates on more than one occasion, simply by attending to and presenting the scientific evidence. Though I respect the ethical argument for not eating animals, my issue with animal protein has never been about animal welfare, only the evidence as it pertains to human health, and various activists have critiqued me for taking that position. Certain advocates of vegan or vegetarian diets have shown that they would rather ignore or deny the evidence obtained by experimental laboratory-animal studies, even when that evidence on health happens to align with their larger cause of not harming and killing animals.

Of course, I have faced much more criticism and petulance from the other side of the debate. As I've written about before, at a 1989 World Congress of Nutrition conference in Seoul, South Korea, during a presentation of my research, a highly influential researcher named Vernon Young, a professor at MIT in food science and nutrition, exclaimed from the audience, "Colin, you're talking about good food. Don't take it away from us!" The food he was talking about, of course, was animal-protein-based food, the food I myself had adored for the first decades of my life, and the food that was the livelihood of my dairy-farming family.

Had Young critiqued my presentation on the basis of the science, it would have sparked a more positive and fruitful exchange, and maybe we would have inched another increment closer to Truth and Wisdom. As it turned out, his actual critique was far more illuminating. It illuminated what has been the central problem of nutrition science forever: it is too often entangled with value judgments about "good" or "bad" food that have nothing to do with evidence. Where do these value judgments come from? They're *supposed* to come from nutrition science, and in an ideal world, they would. However, experience indicates otherwise. The factors that contribute to our idea of what is and is not "good food" are many. Religious, environmental, and ethical considerations come into play; class and culture are undeniable indicators of dietary preference; and foods long associated with wealth and homeland are hard to dethrone, even if evidence suggests they cause disease. And then of course there's tastes.

Clearly, many of the value judgments we attach to foods are not the products of pure science, and it would be naïve to assume that science itself is always able to rise above these judgments. But that has not stopped the production of "evidence" that reinforces those judgments, for when it comes to powerful, popular food industries, there is no shortage of cash on hand to fund favorable studies.

Presumably Vernon Young did not consider himself to be a poor scientist, but he was certainly guilty of putting the cart (his version of "good" food) before the horse (nutrition science). And unfortunately, as he and many like him have taken that attitude into the most influential spaces of nutrition science, the consequences have been severe. To give just one highly damaging example, in 2002 Young served as chair of the macronutrients subcommittee on the Food and Nutrition Board (FNB), which was responsible for establishing, for the first time, an "upper safe limit" (UL) for dietary protein. They set it at a shockingly high 35 percent of total calorie intake, a number that was and remains scientifically unjustified, terribly damaging to human health, and thus, frankly, unconscionable. This recommendation, now widely established, was not even supported with evidence in the body of the report. The recommended daily allowance—an estimate first made by the same FNB in 1943 and revisited every five years since, which measures how much the body needs, on average, to maintain optimum health—recommends that 10 percent of calorie intake should come from dietary protein.

The UL of 35 percent dietary protein is also lacking in practical usefulness. One would have to consume an inordinate amount of animal-based protein to reach this threshold. The difference between a diet containing the recommended 10 percent of calories from protein and a diet containing the upper limit of 35 percent of calories from protein is biologically massive. The former could be achieved by eating an exclusively plant-based diet (plants contain at least 8–10 percent protein), while the latter can only be achieved by eating a nearly carnivorous diet. By endorsing both, we endorse neither. In effect, the recommendation becomes meaningless—have as much protein as you want! This recommendation has the dual effect of protecting industry and giving consumers a feeling of false security.

Of course, the science is less forgiving. The science, which I will discuss further in the following chapters—and which you can, of course, find in greater detail in my previous books—makes it clear that a diet containing 35 percent of calories from protein produces radically different health outcomes than a diet containing 10 percent of calories from protein. The evidence is clear:

1. chronic disease risk increases with even small intakes of animal-based protein;
2. eating more animal-based foods is associated with eating fewer disease-protective whole plant foods;
3. plant-based foods provide all the protein that is needed; and
4. there are numerous biological mechanisms, as discovered in laboratory-animal studies, to explain the damaging effect of eating more animal-based foods and fewer plant-based foods.

Increasing dietary protein intake to just 20 percent, much less 35 percent, has been shown to increase* a range of serious health problems, including cancer, with each successive percentage increase associated with an increase in response, commonly referred to as a dose-response.[1]

Two members of the FNB committee that set this 35 percent upper-limit recommendation are friends of mine. When I questioned them after reading the news release, they seemed unaware that the committee had even established that conclusion. One of those friends, Joe Rodricks, a long-time senior

---

* Keep in mind that the observed increases in disease risk in population studies are not due only to animal protein; with the consumption of more animal protein, other nutrient intakes also shift significantly. Collectively, these changes have a very substantial effect.

scientist and administrator at the FDA, initially and understandably became defensive about the supporting data for this limit (or rather, the lack of supporting data), but finally admitted to me, when I challenged him, "Colin, you know I don't know anything about nutrition." His area of specialty, as I did know, was actually toxicology! My other friend and colleague on the committee claimed to have never even seen the 35 percent figure published in the news release, telling me he must have missed it because there was so much material to read as the committee was winding up its business. Given that the 35 percent upper limit is highlighted in the opening sentence of the press release,[2] this raises a number of questions. Namely, who wrote this disease-producing recommendation, and when did they write it? How much input did they receive from the other members of the committee? How responsible were the FNB's leaders, and how impactful were their industry connections?

And yes, there were industry connections. The chair of the FNB, Cutberto Garza, was, to say the least of our contentious relationship, an acquaintance of mine. He served a total of twelve years as the director of the Division of Nutritional Sciences at Cornell (my academic home), and throughout that time his arguments often aligned with dairy industry interests. On one such occasion, at an International Congress of Nutrition meeting in Quebec, he argued on behalf of Nestlé Corporation—the biggest food company in the world, which has played a central role in the dairy industry ever since its founding in 1866.[3] On another, he and the federal agencies that established the Dietary Guidelines Advisory Committee, of which he was also chair, were successfully sued for undisclosed conflicts of interest by the Physicians Committee for Responsible Medicine, who argued that six of the eleven members (including Garza) were unacceptably associated with the dairy and egg industries. For Garza himself, the lead agency failed to disclose personal compensation that was far in excess of the reporting threshold set by the agency.* As for Vernon Young, following his chairing of the above-cited 2002 macronutrients subcommittee of the Food and Nutrition Board, he served on Nestlé's board of directors.

---

* Told to me by the attorney of record in that case.

These examples only barely scratch the surface of the food industry's profound influence over nutrition science. At a 2018 presentation before the New Jersey Academy of Nutrition and Dietetics, I began by polling the 300 clinical dietitians in attendance on their views on the upper safe limit for dietary protein. A strong majority (70–80 percent) recognized and seemingly accepted the 35 percent upper limit—more than three times what the science supports! And these same dietitians are now responsible for working with the public on matters of nutrition? Though not willfully so, many well-intentioned professional dietitians are woefully misinformed. Can you blame them? Their profession was fed these lies by a widely regarded and authoritative institution. Even more frightening is the fact that the FNB's established UL has a foundational impact on the development of public policy. Every day it harms the health of millions of Americans, including thirty million schoolchildren in the School Lunch Program and its affiliates, and eight million participants in the Women, Infants, and Children program.*

But I believe it would be unwise to characterize these examples as outliers. To do so is to underestimate the expansiveness and severity of the problem the field of nutrition faces. The resistance I have experienced throughout my career, as well as the heated debates over dietary preferences that have become completely normal, are symptomatic of a more fundamental crisis. To use a disease metaphor, these "tumors" are not *local* in their origins and treatments, but *constitutional*. They prove, as well as any other example, that our society's narrative on nutrition is fractured in a way that increases opportunities for exploitation, and that our leaders in this field are the chief exploiters themselves.

As such, the time for change *within* these systems is past, for they no longer function effectively. We cannot sit idly by and wait for their redemption. If they were capable of such self-repair, if the process were functional, then the recommended UL of 35 percent for dietary protein would have been challenged nearly twenty years ago. Upon closer examination of the evidence, it would have been dismissed as unscientific. The industry affiliations of its authors would have been publicized, even subjected to legal scrutiny.

---

* This program provides to its participants, among other services, supplemental food and information about healthy eating.

But such checks and balances are impossible when the leadership of both the FNB and the Dietary Guidelines Advisory Committee of the USDA are the same, as was the case under Garza. If our institutions functioned effectively, one person never would have been allowed to simultaneously hold both positions, one that makes nutrient-specific recommendations (FNB) and one that translates those recommendations into guidelines for total dietary consumption—particularly when that person had recently failed to disclose his ties to the dairy industry.

CULTIVATING CONFUSION

With this and many other examples of mixed messages, bias, and deception among professionals, how could we expect a well-informed, healthy public? And government recommendations like the one above are not our only source of nutrition information. We also receive messages on nutrition from various forms of media: lifestyle books, blogs, magazines, podcasts, and advertising. It seems to me that most of the public's nutrition "schooling" today involves the accumulation of conflicting information, but few to no skills to sort through and judge the veracity of that information.

Have we ever been taught discernment? According to a 2013 cross-sectional study[4] in which researchers used questionnaires to study "the nutrition-related knowledge, attitudes, and behaviors among Head Start teachers" in Texas, the answer is no. The reason Head Start teachers are especially good subjects for a study like this is because they work on the front lines of early childhood education and serve low-income communities that disproportionately struggle with nutrition-related diseases. Moreover, Head Start centers around the country have made teaching healthy eating a high priority. This is reflected in the attitudes of the surveyed teachers, the vast majority of whom (92.7 percent) agreed with the statement "Learning the relationship between food and health is important." Although I question the degree to which they believe nutrition is important, for the reasons discussed in Part I—as a result of institutional beliefs, we as a society do not fully grasp nutrition's role in disease formation and treatment—the point stands: these are people with good intentions and a desire to understand the fundamentals of nutrition. Unfortunately, more than four out of five Head Start teachers were either unsure or agreed with the statement "It's hard to know which nutrition information to believe," and just under four out of five were either overweight or obese. Basically, the vast majority of them are confused about nutrition and their health proves it. So does the rest of the questionnaire. When asked five elementary questions to test their knowledge of nutrition (e.g., which has more calories: protein, carbohydrate, or fat?), only 3 percent answered four of the questions correctly. *None* could answer all five questions correctly.

I would suggest that Head Start teachers are normal in both their intentions and their confusion. They reflect the general public of today, and unless we change course, they will reflect the general public of tomorrow. The frightening truth is that there are many powerful interests that would like to see these trends continue. A confused consumer is a gullible consumer, and gullible consumers fatten the wallets and purses of the food, pharmaceutical, and supplement industries.

In a 2015 *Public Health* article,[5] New Zealand researcher Janet Hoek describes how this same phenomenon applied to the tobacco industry of the 1950s and '60s, whose "strategy of undermining scientists by challenging their credibility and motivation, and presenting opposing 'expert' views, successfully generated confusion among smokers." The logic of Big Tobacco then, and of the food industry today, is simple: it is easier (and more effective) to confuse the public than to defend a poisonous product.

Likewise, powerful industries can't convince us to *entirely* stop caring about our health. The buying public will always want information to improve their health and their family's health, at least to a certain extent. Therefore, the best option that remains for industry is to encourage confusion until eventually our good sense is completely eroded by decision fatigue. The more authors, speakers, and internet health gurus there are to compete for your attention, the better the marketing environment. The more often that minute details, like the focus on some would-be nutrient or phytochemical, are blown out of proportion, and honest science distorted or robbed of its context, the easier it is for industry to repackage our bad habits and sell them to us in the newest quick-and-easy diet product—made *just* for us! Part of this problem arises from the fact that this information may be reasonably or partially correct, but only when isolated from context (and this is not the way Nature works). As a result, it is difficult for a scientifically untrained person to know what to believe.

It seems industry understands this aspect of human psychology better than we do. They recognize and rely on the cognitive biases and rationalizations that take over when confusion reigns, as illustrated by oft-repeated phrases like "*everyone* has to die at some point" and "*anything* is bad for you, depending on how you look at it" and "*everything* in moderation." The first is true, but misses the point entirely—good nutrition is not about indefinitely avoiding death, but about living a healthy, fulfilling life. The second is a fallacious appeal to extremes—it pays lip service to everything, while saying nothing. And the third takes wishful thinking to a new level, as if even heroin might be healthy in moderation. What these three sayings have in common is that they all reflect our resignation in the face of so much conflicting nutrition information, they all reinforce the status quo, and they're all beautiful melodies in the ears of marketing executives.

THE CONTROVERSY OF THE WFPB DIET

Until we disrupt the patterns described above, the science of nutrition will remain clogged, cluttered, and underutilized. And as we incorporate new labels into our panoply of *-isms*, piling atop the already existing *vegetarianism, veganism, carnivorism, pescatarianism, fruitarianism*, and more, these labels will likely create more confusion than clarity, if the past is anything to go by. "Whole food, plant-based" is yet another label in danger of abuse by hucksters, but I would argue that it is the most desirable yet, precisely because it, and the diet it describes, disrupts the trends introduced in this chapter.

It is disruptive, first of all, because it challenges the popular concept of dieting as something short term, to be endured and suffered through, hopefully with some weight loss earned as a result. The WFPB diet is more of a dietary *lifestyle*. It offers guidelines for a long and healthy life, not a punishing shortcut to superficial change.

The second, more pertinent reason the WFPB dietary lifestyle is disruptive is that it forces us to reckon with long-held value judgments about what is and is not "good food." It does not condemn the many factors that determine an individual's dietary preferences, but it does raise questions about them. I'm reminded once again of Vernon Young and his plea that I not take the foods he enjoyed away from him, and also of an old friend and colleague of mine, Professor Dick Warner. Raised by a butcher father, he completed his graduate studies at Cornell before taking a faculty position in animal nutrition. His particular focus was the nutritional properties of animal-based protein, and he was a significant person in my career, not least for his guidance as cochair on my PhD research advisory committee from 1958 to 1961. When I returned to my faculty position at Cornell with a greater focus on human nutrition, fourteen years later, our interests in animal protein had diverged greatly, but our interactions, though few, remained pleasant all the same.

A few years after my return, Dick visited my office to discuss a personal issue. He had undergone a couple of heart bypass operations and wanted to know more about my research. At the time, I'd been hosting yearly lectures in my class from Dr. Caldwell Esselstyn Jr., who discussed his clinical experiences successfully treating heart patients using a low-fat WFPB diet, and so I invited Dick to attend. Dick did so and eventually committed to making moderate changes to his diet. After one year, he'd decreased his fat intake to 10–12 percent of calories and felt somewhat better as a result, but he achieved this mainly by replacing other meats with lean turkey. You see, he wanted to improve his health, but did not want to give up meat.

After attending a second lecture from Esselstyn a year later, Dick pulled me aside at a party to discuss something that had been on his mind. A devoted man of faith, he reminded me of a couple passages from the Old Testament. He quoted Genesis 1:29, in which God said, "I give you every seed-bearing plant on the face of the whole earth and every tree that has fruit with seed in it [which] will be yours for food," but then later relented in Genesis 9:3 after the flood: "Everything that lives and moves will be food for you. Just as I gave you the green plants, I now give you everything." Dick interpreted this second passage to mean that he was abiding by the wishes of God by eating meat.

Now, I am by no means informed in these matters, but neither am I disparaging Dick's faith. I knew that Dick, besides being a leader in his Methodist church, was a very principled man in other areas of his life. In fact, he held the distinguished position of university ombudsman, an office that oversees individual rights and helps to resolve disputes. Once he phoned to tell me that he had overheard comments on campus about some of my more radical views, but wanted to let me know that I had his full support and that he respected my integrity. What strikes me most about his story is not his biblical research, but that so many different factors competed to influence his diet: personal health considerations, scientific evidence, and religious interpretation.

His choices were intensely personal, and whose aren't? Whether you believe animals have been put on this earth for our use, advocate for animal rights, or occupy some middle ground, the food we eat is of personal importance. I understand and respect the freedom of people to choose. Dick Warner's choice was different from mine, but I remember him as a personally kind and caring soul.

The WFPB diet is disruptive because it instigates the kind of reckoning that Dick Warner's story illustrates. Its first concern is not with choice, but with science, and so it cannot avoid calling our choices into question, even choices of great sensitivity. The evidence against animal protein is not evidence against your faith or taste buds, but evidence that moves us closer to clarity in the science of nutrition.

And I believe that this is the third and most important reason that the WFPB diet is disruptive to the trends discussed in this chapter. Unlike a vegan diet, which is also disruptive to the meat and dairy industries, the WFPB diet threatens to disrupt the most pervasive characteristic of the status quo in nutrition today: confusion. In the simplicity of its message and the strength of its supporting evidence, it offers clarity.

Perhaps this clarity doesn't seem like a big deal, but it is. As long as the status quo tends toward confusion, as it does now, the pursuit of clarity will be a significant source of hope for the confused consumer. And when confusion is normal, any step toward clarity is a form of *protest*. The confusion we tend toward can be seen from top to bottom, in the work of nutrition professionals, the Head Start program, and everywhere in between. Nutrition is confusing in great part because so many of the most influential actors and leaders in this discipline are themselves confused. Their interpretation of the scientific evidence is influenced by the blatant corruption of industry, sure, but also by personal biases—though these biases themselves may have developed out of extended corporate influence on the public narrative. Like the rest of society, nutrition professionals are swayed by a wide array of considerations that figure into our value judgments about food. We are no less susceptible to defensiveness, a stubborn attachment to certain foods, and contradictory beliefs about what is and is not "good" food. In these ways, we professionals feed from the same trough of confusion as the public.

Said another way: when the majority of voices in industry, academia, and policy are pulling us in the same direction, toward confusion, then anything that promotes clarity is a direct challenge and *is* controversial. And anything that upends the "good food" narratives so dear to our hearts, narratives that often pollute our thinking at a subconscious level, will be controversial.

There is one example in the field of nutrition, above all others, that testifies to the public's confusion, our susceptibility to such narratives, and the difficulty of change. It is the example of animal protein. Much as cancer research past and present exemplifies our society's disconnect between malnutrition and disease, the example of animal protein shines a spotlight on the confusion in nutrition as we know it and promises tremendous room for growth.

CHAPTER FIVE

THE CULT OF ANIMAL PROTEIN

This cold night will turn us all to fools and madmen.
—William Shakespeare

I n 1839 researchers discovered that dogs in a laboratory would die if
their food was missing a certain vital substance.[1-3] This was the first
discovery of its kind, excluding that of oxygen, and it gave rise to the
concept of essential nutrients—those nutrients that we must consume to
maintain health, because our bodies cannot make them (e.g., fat, carbohydrates, vitamins, and minerals). So important was this newly discovered
substance that it was named *protein*, from the Greek word *proteios,* meaning "of prime importance." A promising baptism, but minor compared to
what would come.

Early on, the Dutch organic chemist Gerhard Mulder (1802–1880) described protein as "unquestionably the most important of all known substances in the organic kingdom. Without it, no life appears possible on our planet. Through the use of protein, the chief phenomena of life are produced."[4] Soon after, Justus von Liebig (1803–1873), the German founder of agricultural chemistry and organic chemistry, described protein as "the stuff of life itself." Liebig is arguably the most prodigious biological scientist in all of history; an extraordinary 700 students studied under Liebig at an institution that still bears his name. Four decades later, his student, Professor Carl von Voit of Germany (1831–1908), echoed his sentiments when making recommendations for protein consumption. Tremendously influential in his own right, and commonly described as the father of dietetics and nutrition, Voit recommended a diet with a large amount of protein—substantially more than was justified by his own research. In that research, he observed that 52 grams per day of protein was enough for good health, but he ended up recommending more than twice as much—118 grams per day—as did seven of his colleagues (whose recommendations ranged from 100–134 g/day).[5,6] And when these early nutrition authorities spoke of protein in general, what they really meant was *animal protein*.

Now, if you're feeling generous, you might give these towering authorities the benefit of the doubt. You might speculate that perhaps they never considered the possibility of overconsumption, and so they made what they thought were generous recommendations, hoping that even those consuming less would still get enough. Alternatively, you might call their exaggerated recommendations what they were: unjustified and reckless (if not irresponsible). Regardless, it seems clear that they were swept up in the hype surrounding protein. This is unsurprising, given how hyperbolic much of the early commentary surrounding protein was. One of Voit's students, Max Rubner (1854–1932), famed for his work on energy metabolism (and for coining the word *calorie*), claimed that protein was the "interchange of civilization itself." In another case, documents suggest that an English medical adviser in India named Major McCay favored men of the Bengali tribe over other indigenous peoples because they consumed the most protein.[7] Those who consumed less protein were described as being of an "effeminate nature." Likewise, he described the "inferior races" of the world as those that did not consume enough animal protein, as did H. H. Mitchell, a highly influential American nutrition researcher who developed the standard equation for determining the nutritional value of protein from animal sources, as discussed later in this book.[8]

Whatever the motives of their champions, these early attitudes have had tremendous consequences. These men were, after all, the most influential figures in the field, and their intellectual descendants are beyond counting. To give you an idea of how far their influence has spread, consider another student of Voit's, W. O. Atwater (1844–1907). Atwater went on to found the first nutrition programs at the USDA—programs that still, more than a century later, influence the conduct of the organization's US Dietary Guidelines Advisory Committee. One of today's professional honors in nutritional science is the annual W. O. Atwater memorial lecture, hosted by the USDA.

This lineage, in and of itself, is not the problem. So long as the field could evolve, it wouldn't matter so much whether early enthusiasm for protein was excessive. Unfortunately, the field has shown a stubborn inability to move beyond that early enthusiasm, despite a great deal of subsequent research showing that enthusiasm to be excessive both then and now. Since Atwater, through the establishment of food and nutrition programs during World War II, to modern times, USDA nutrition scientists have continued to beat the drums for high-protein foods, especially animal-based foods (meat, dairy, and eggs). The "Basic 7 Food Groups" guidelines introduced in 1943 recommended daily servings of two to three glasses of milk for adults and three to four for children; three to five eggs; at least one serving of meat, cheese, fish, or poultry; modest servings of vegetables, fruits, whole-grain breads; and, occasionally, dried beans, peas, or peanuts.[9] These recommendations, in principle, are not that different from today's, except now the USDA favors even higher levels of dietary protein that can only be met with greater consumption of animal protein—recall the upper limit of 35 percent discussed in chapter four.

The pattern of overconsumption set by Carl von Voit and his contemporaries in the late 1800s has held steady, despite many consequences, and shows little sign of slowing down. Americans continue to eat protein far in excess of the amount proven to maintain optimal health (17–18 percent of calories, versus the 8–10 percent recommended and the 5–6 percent required to balance nitrogen losses). Though different metrics have been used to express protein requirements and recommendations (e.g., grams per kilogram of body weight, grams per day), the most appropriate metric expresses protein as a *proportion of total calories*, which references the kind of diet being used. Recommendations of specific quantities should be avoided: they only present more confusion, infer isolated and independent activities of protein that do not differentiate the nutritional activities of animal and plant sources, and encourage protein supplementation.

The primacy of animal protein, compared to both plant protein and other nutrients, has become so normalized that it's almost compulsive. It is never far from our minds, whether conscious or subconscious. This is why nearly everyone on a plant-based diet has been questioned about where they get their protein, rather than their vitamin B_{12} or any other nutrient of note. Protein is king, and animal protein is the noblest king of all—the just, disciplined, and virile king that every peasant dreams of. In its ascendency to that position, it has infected our scientific measurements, our language, and our policy. We continue to bend over backward to maintain the outsized celebration granted to animal protein from its earliest days—and rationalize it as superior to plant protein.

MEASURING ANIMAL PROTEIN: A "HIGH-QUALITY" SMOKESCREEN

The disciples of animal protein often assert that it has greater "nutritive value" than the proteins of plants. This concept of nutritive value is frequently assumed, though scientists have different ways of describing it. The more common description, and likely the way you've heard this concept in your own life, is that animal protein is "high quality." I will use these terms—"quality" and "nutritive value"—interchangeably throughout this chapter. But to understand the origins of this belief about animal protein's superiority, we need to go back to the beginning.

From the first decades after protein's discovery through today, many scientists have sought to develop objective methods for determining the relative value of different proteins, including both plant and animal proteins. This is a perfectly understandable goal, but one that has turned out to be deeply flawed in practice, because the favored methods have been used primarily to reinforce the value of our favored foods, particularly animal-based foods.

The earliest and perhaps most rudimentary of these methods was the "protein efficiency ratio" (PER). A food's PER is found by dividing gain in body mass by protein intake. That is, it measures the efficiency of different proteins in promoting body growth. And although mostly used by farmers and agriculture researchers rather than in human health, PER is worth considering because it reflects how our fetish for protein carries over to inferences about human health.

The PER method focuses on maximizing growth (the proteins with the highest PER values result in the greatest amount of salable product and profit). When it comes to human health, however, the flaw of measuring nutritive value in this way is obvious. It assumes that the *fastest* rate of growth is also the *optimal* rate of growth.

The more widely used measure of protein quality throughout much of the twentieth century was a protein's "biological value" (BV). Developed by a University of Illinois professor of animal husbandry named H. H. Mitchell in 1924,[10] BV is used to describe the proportion of nitrogen retained in the body upon consumption of a given protein. In essence, it is supposed to measure the *efficiency of use* of various proteins. It assumes that the nitrogen retained in the body is being put to good use—an assumption that, even today, is unjustified by the scientific literature. The specific bias of H. H. Mitchell toward animal protein is also impossible to ignore. Much like Major McCay working in India, Mitchell viewed protein consumption as a determinant of racial status. In one account, he referred to some races as "inferior" because they did not consume what he considered to be enough animal-based protein.[8,10] Although BV, like PER, is not often directly cited in discussions about the importance of protein for human health, I present it here because, historically, it generated a popular understanding of animal-based protein as superior to plant-based protein.

More recently, the "amino acid score" (AAS) was developed. To understand this measure, it's important to know that proteins are built from long chains of amino acids, like beads on a string. After a person eats proteins, the body breaks them down into individual amino acids in the intestine, before reassembling them after intestinal absorption to form new proteins for itself. The AAS measures how faithfully the arrangement of amino acids in various food proteins matches the arrangement of amino acids the body reassembles to use. Animal-based proteins contain the amounts and proportions of amino acids most similar to ours (unsurprisingly, being that we're animals, too), whereas plant-based proteins differ. As a result, AAS proponents assume the proteins in animal foods allow for more efficient use, giving rise to the aforementioned idea that they are "high quality." Generally speaking, they contain in the right proportion and in the right order a set of nine amino acids that are considered essential to consume because we cannot synthesize them. (Incidentally, if we were to take this measure to its logical conclusion, we would have to conclude that the "highest-quality" protein is derived from *human flesh*—try serving that for Thanksgiving!) Individual plant proteins, which lack one or more of the nine essential amino acids, are thus called "low quality."

At its core, measuring protein quality by AAS is not so different from the PER and BV measures that preceded it. Although AAS is more specific and technically impressive, it ultimately measures the same thing: *efficiency* and *usability*. This long-held preference for efficiency and usability is the defining pattern that, at every turn, has determined our preferred valuation methods. There are, of course, more methods than just these three. A food's "protein digestibility–corrected amino acid score" likewise measures amino acids, but also considers the amount of amino acids absorbed into the blood from the intestine, essentially tweaking the AAS method by eliminating one level of variation occurring during digestion. Additionally, there are measures of nitrogen balance and net protein utilization.[11] No need to further describe them, because they all rest on the same wrongheaded assumption: that the more efficiently the protein is used in the body, after digestion and absorption into the blood, the greater will be the health outcome, and so the greater the "quality" of that protein. The often-ignored, uncomfortable fact is that this assumption is unfounded. Just as it makes no sense to assume that faster growth equals greater health, it makes no sense to assume that greater absorption or greater retention is preferable. To make this assumption, we'd need to be confident that the nitrogen and/or amino acids retained are all being put to good use, and we simply cannot prove this.

We also cannot focus, as these specific measures do, solely on the specific effects of the protein in animal-based foods; we must look at the wider effects those foods have on human health. Animal protein, as food, is packaged with many other substances, including questionable ones like cholesterol and saturated fat. Indeed, odd as it may sound, *no known health risks at all* figure into our assessment of protein value. Never mind that along with increased body growth, the accumulation of protein in our bodies may also increase the rate of cancer growth, serum cholesterol levels, and cardiovascular disease risk. Given the massive and ongoing toll of people killed or disabled by these pernicious diseases, you might think we would take a more nuanced approach to our assessment of protein quality.

Even the presumed benefits of animal protein may be misunderstood. Take growth, for example. After being shown that "high-quality" animal protein produced a faster rate of growth in pigs and rats, it was inferred that the same would be true in children. This is probably correct. And of course, growth is particularly important for children. Besides being an essential part of health, robust growth conveys the impression of superiority and strength in many cultures around the world. However, early rate of body growth does not necessarily translate into greater adult height and physical prowess. Our ultimate height is more closely related to genetic predisposition, though early childhood diseases and other influences can also reduce attained adult height. Absent these problems, which are more common in impoverished parts of the world, childhood diets without animal protein do support equal attainment of healthy adult height. Moreover, faster rate of childhood growth caused by "high-quality" animal-based protein does not necessarily mean *healthier* adults. Indeed, consuming "high-quality" animal protein increases growth hormone, resulting in earlier sexual maturation, higher levels of sex hormones, and increased risk of cancer of the reproductive organs.[12-17] I find it scandalous that these well-documented adverse effects have been omitted from our valuation of protein quality for so many decades.

In my own research program in the 1970s and 1980s on experimental rats, discussed in greater depth in chapter nine as well as in *The China Study*, we repeatedly established the ability of higher consumption of the milk-based protein casein to dramatically increase a growth hormone associated with increased cancer development.[18,19] In contrast, high levels of a "low-quality" wheat protein had the opposite effect. Due to its "deficiency" in the amino acid lysine, the wheat protein *prevented* cancer development. (We know that the missing lysine was responsible for this change because when lysine was restored, cancer growth resumed to the same level as for the casein.[20]) In other words, the animal-based protein increased cancer growth while the plant-based protein in its original form did not, until its amino acid profile was "improved" to the level of its animal-based counterpart.

THE LANGUAGE OF ANIMAL PROTEIN

Based on these measures of nutritive value, many lay dieters and on-the-ground health professionals perpetuate the notion that animal protein is "high quality." It's hard to blame them; after all, who wouldn't want evidence-based methods to objectively determine quality? Whether we're aware of it or not, most of us find comfort and security in measures of quality that can be quantified, even when those measurements are deeply flawed. The more precise our quantification, the more we feel like authentic scientists, and the more it appeals to our numbers-fixated society, even when *qualitative* analysis is more appropriate.

In any case, the biological values we assign to proteins are not entirely useless. We have just become accustomed to reading them incorrectly, through more than a century of schooling. For example, the lower values assigned to plant protein are telling us something useful. When presented with the more limited amino acid profiles of plant proteins, it seems that our bodies are able to control their use in a way they biologically prefer. This is a good thing, not a deficiency. Yet we have misread the lower body-growth responses plant-based proteins produce as a design flaw. Conversely, we have misread the potency of animal-based proteins as potential for good health, and efficiency as excellence. "The more the better," we repeat again and again. Even though we know that the average person on a plant-based diet is less likely to be overweight, develop cancer of the reproductive organs (among others), and develop cardiovascular disease than the average omnivore, we continue to misread these "values."

I suggest that these mistakes are dictated by faulty patterns of thought, and that our thoughts are reflected in and further cultured by misguided language. Therefore, in order to move beyond these mistakes, it would be helpful to move beyond the language that brought us here in the first place. Until we are able to do so, progress will be hampered.

Besides the "high-quality" label, there are several examples among health authorities of how our language continues to hold us back. Consider the International Agency for Research on Cancer (IARC) of the United Nations' World Health Organization (WHO), which in 2015 labeled processed meat as carcinogenic and red meat as "probably carcinogenic." Not surprisingly, given how influential this organization is, this message made major news around the world. My own take on the research that gave rise to this labeling was somewhat different than the researchers' and how it was reported on by the media: I am less concerned by the carcinogenicity of processed meat specifically than I am by the cancer-promoting role of all sources of animal protein, the corresponding lack of plant foods, and their complex interplay.*

Having lectured twice at IARC, I can assure you that these scientists are reluctant to believe that nutrition might play any role whatsoever in cancer causation. Their official purpose is to pass judgment on possible chemical carcinogens *in* food, not the food itself. In fact, even this 2015 announcement came forty to fifty years after it was first reported that meat might be associated with increased cancer risk.[21–23] Not exactly cutting edge. And so, I was somewhat surprised and a little skeptical of the 2015 announcement.

Consider the greater context: in a 2018 update on those findings, the IARC reminded the public that "red meat contains *proteins* of high *biological value*, as well as important micronutrients such as B-vitamins, iron . . . and zinc" (their emphasis). Why would IARC go out of its way to sing the praises of a food that they themselves have labeled "probably carcinogenic," when all the available evidence suggests a diet *free* of red meat could provide the same nutrients, if not more safely and effectively? Besides their long-time concern

---

* A note on the processed meat specification here: the statistical distinction between processed and unprocessed meat was minor and likely of little or no importance. The effect observed for processed meat fell just over the borderline for statistical significance, while the effect of unprocessed meat fell just beneath the same borderline. This enabled IARC to somewhat downplay the deleterious effects of unprocessed meat.

for chemical carcinogens and long-time disregard for nutrition, perhaps it's also because they're unable to see beyond the so-called biological value of animal-based protein, even when contradictions arise?

Such mixed messages are not uncommon. In a 2017 paper on red meat intake and chronic kidney disease, the abstract's first sentence states that "red meat is an important dietary source of high biological value protein," but then goes on to suggest that "limiting the intake of red meat in patients with chronic kidney diseases (CKD) . . . may slow the progression of kidney disease" and may be "a good strategy to reduce CV [cardiovascular disease] risk" that often accompanies CKD.[24] All this in the same abstract! I can't help but pity the strain that these scientists are clearly struggling under, torn between their own findings and century-old dogma. The mental acrobatics would exhaust anyone. As with the IARC report, I ask again, why do these scientists continue to cling to the outdated terminology of "higher biological value"? Surely the proteins with the highest biological value would be those that come from foods that *prevent and reverse** kidney disease, *prevent and reverse* cardiovascular disease, and are *provably* anti-cancerous, rather than probably carcinogenic? There are hundreds of research reports from influential institutions and highly respected research groups that continue to parrot the same flawed "high quality" story. It is deeply embedded within our language, and so deeply embedded in our beliefs.

The impact of our misused and selective language is profound. We justify our bad nutritional habits with positive concepts like high nitrogen retention, efficiency of use, rate of body growth, efficiency of production, and enhanced activities of enzymes that detoxify toxic chemicals, while consistently omitting the negative ones like high serum cholesterol, lesser

---

* A remarkable case study of the WFPB diet's ability to treat chronic kidney disease has been recently published by my son Tom in the prestigious *British Medical Journal*.[25] The paper describes how stage III CKD, diabetes, hypertension, and obesity were substantially reversed in a sixty-nine-year-old man consuming a low-animal-protein, WFPB diet for 4.5 months. His insulin medication was reduced more than 50 percent, most of his twelve drugs were eliminated, his body weight decreased by more than seventy pounds, and his glomerular filtration rate—a critical measure of kidney function—increased by 64 percent. These WFPB diet effects, consistent with those found in several other studies on low-protein diets, some going back as far as a century,[26] offer a tremendous opportunity to today's nearly 800 million people with CKD worldwide.[27]

physical performance, increased cancer risk, cardiovascular disease, tissue degeneration with age, metabolic acidosis, formation of reactive oxidative species, and high serum estrogen and growth hormone. And it's high time we stopped.

In short, I hope never to hear the words "high quality" associated with animal protein again. Let's call it what it is: a myth.

THE POLICY OF ANIMAL PROTEIN: FEEDING THE WORLD?

In addition to its infiltration into the methods and language of science and public perception, animal protein has also benefited from decades of misguided policy. At least since the time of Voit's early recommendations, we have let our fear of protein deficiency cloud our judgment. This fear has even become a matter of international concern, as evidenced by a number of global health policy efforts since the early years of my career.

In the 1930s, a severe form of undernourishment named kwashiorkor was described for the first time in the scientific literature.[28] It came to be most closely associated with protein deficiency, which dominated the focus of both individuals and institutions over the rest of the century. Decades after kwashiorkor's discovery, the Institute of Nutrition of Central America and Panama (INCAP) was founded to address undernourishment globally—specifically, to help resolve childhood malnutrition by ensuring adequate protein consumption.[29] Funded by the Ford and Rockefeller foundations[30] and initially directed by perhaps the best-known nutrition scientist in the world during the second half of the twentieth century, Professor Nevin Scrimshaw of MIT, INCAP quickly became one of the leading childhood nutrition institutes in the world.

As well-meaning as the individuals and institutions involved may have been, their exaggerated focus on protein remains questionable. Even the condition kwashiorkor itself, and its prevalence, might have been exaggerated. During my early research in the Philippines on childhood malnourishment, I too described kwashiorkor as a protein deficiency, until I began asking around and couldn't find any physicians who had seen clear evidence of the disease. A few other commenters similarly questioned the emphasis placed on protein in the condition.[31,32] Nevertheless, the extreme malnourishment of children in the developing world was passed on as evidence of a "protein gap,"[2] adding enthusiasm and urgency to calls for greater protein consumption.

It was generally accepted that cow's milk protein would best serve to plug the protein gap, but it was expensive.[33] Therefore, Scrimshaw and his associates developed a cereal-based alternative that combined several plant-based proteins (corn flour, soy flour, cottonseed meal, and Torula yeast[33]) to mimic the amino acid profile of cow's milk. The fact that this alternative was plant-based is not the important point and was only due to cost. INCAP did not advocate for whole plant foods, but rather a concoction of plant fragments that might closely approximate the glorious amino acid profile of cow's milk. This product was named, somewhat unoriginally, INCAPARINA. In the fifty years since its creation, nutrition scientists have tweaked and tested the concoction many times, and its use has been incredibly widespread. As recently as 2010, 80 percent of children in Guatemala were still being fed INCAPARINA in their first year of life to prevent protein deficiency.[34]

Unfortunately, these efforts have been largely ineffective. In 2010, Ricardo Bresanni, former director of the Division of Agricultural Sciences and Food at INCAP,*c wrote a commentary on INCAP's history of more than fifty years.[33] Though the report sings the praises of healthy, plant-based supplements in general, it offers no conclusive evidence that INCAPARINA has benefited malnourished children, hedging that "it is difficult to know the precise impact that Incaparina has had on the elimination of malnutrition in the general population, because economic status has been improving concurrently. Moreover, solving these multifaceted, complex problems with one solution is too much to be expected." These concluding remarks seem balanced and fair. And, on the final point, I agree wholeheartedly: expecting a simple solution (protein supplements) to solve a complex problem (widespread malnutrition) is an absurd idea. But that just raises the same question,

---

* Incidentally, I shared an office with Bressani at MIT in 1964–65.

once again: Why has protein deficiency been the central task and focus of INCAP since its founding?

None of this is to say that there wasn't a crisis of malnutrition in the developing world, or that such a crisis doesn't still exist. I am only questioning our methods of dealing with it—in particular the lopsided focus on protein, which has perpetuated the myth of animal protein's value. Through programs like INCAP, that myth has been flung far and wide. In addition to distributing supplemental products, INCAP has also had a tremendous impact on developing "professional expertise" in nutrition. The knock-on effect of this is significant: if INCAP's *particular brand* of professional expertise includes misguided ideas about protein consumption, then those same misguided ideas will be integrated into the "professional expertise" of nutrition and health professionals worldwide, no matter how well-intentioned those professionals may be.

I'm open to alternate interpretations of the history of animal protein and its dominance within the field of nutrition. However, it seems indisputable that this nutrient has enjoyed a long and unusually strong grip on the imaginations of nutrition professionals—and I do mean "imaginations," since in no way does its hallowed status reflect the science. If I'm correct in this interpretation, then what might we expect to see? Decades of international and domestic policy disproportionately concerned with protein deficiency? Nutrition recommendations disproportionately favoring high protein consumption, such as the Food and Nutrition Board's 35 percent upper limit described in chapter four? A clannish mentality in academia, in research funding, even in international aid? A massive protein supplement industry? The incessant question posed to those following a plant-based diet, "Where do you get your protein?"

Sound familiar?

MY RUN-IN WITH ANIMAL PROTEIN

I grew up on a dairy farm where my family produced our own meat, milk, and eggs, and I hunted, fished, and trapped whenever time permitted. For these reasons, I understand the love affair with animal-based protein better than most nutrition scientists ever could. The fascination with animal foods, for me, has always been deeply personal. Perhaps it is even in my DNA; my mom used to proudly say, "My middle name is 'Meat.'" She worked incredibly hard to feed and care for our family, and that included providing a source of animal protein at every meal. Later, when I went to Cornell, my doctoral research focused on how to improve the production of animal-based protein. In sum, I was in deep, and my bias was always *toward* animal protein.

I mention this past only to emphasize how deeply ingrained our beliefs about nutrition can become, how early those habits may be adopted (or rather, how early they may adopt us), and how easy they are to accept without question. I was raised to believe in the value of animal protein, and later educated to accept and share the beliefs of my peers in academia. And though being raised on a dairy farm may have given me a slight head start in this indoctrination, the fact is that my near reverence for animal protein is all too common. Nearly all of us have been raised to believe in the goodness of animal protein, whether we justify it by measures of "nutritive value" or simply by the love of our mothers who put food on the table. This belief is both conscious and subconscious, and its consequences are self-evident. Like so many others, I believed that animal protein was superior to plant protein for the very same reasons I've previously outlined. I hungrily and happily swallowed the "high nutritive value" story. As melodramatic as it may sound, my former life depended on it! Everywhere I turned, I saw more examples of how these measures, and this fundamental belief in the superiority of animal protein, dominated collective thought. I used the BV measure in my doctoral dissertation research, and in teaching my first course on "Feeds and Feeding of Livestock." Even my faculty adviser for my doctoral studies was the son of a lifelong butcher!

My early career work in a childhood nutrition program in the Philippines, funded by the Agency for International Development of the US State Department, was very similar to INCAP's aforementioned work. Like Scrimshaw and his colleagues at MIT, my senior colleague Charlie Engel and I searched for a cheap, plant-based alternative to cow's milk protein to address early childhood malnutrition. Peanuts were our first choice, before concerns arose that they were contaminated with a potent carcinogen, aflatoxin (AF), known to cause liver cancer in laboratory rats.[33] The MIT group had come up against the same problem and experimented with the possibility of chemically removing AF with alkali, but this was not feasible. Later, our group even produced our own plant-based protein supplement, similar to INCAPARINA, called NutriBun (Dr. Engel's formula).

It is especially noteworthy that we were on the same pathway as the MIT group, both in researching the fundamentals of protein function in the laboratory, and in the role of protein in "developing" countries' childhood nutrition programs, given that we ultimately arrived at such different conclusions. Both our groups reflected a broader conversation arising among international nutrition communities about a global protein gap, especially in poor countries, that had to be solved. But while our challenges were similar, it soon became abundantly clear that my evolving interest in protein, both its laboratory-based fundamentals and its practical application, substantially differed from that of the MIT group.

While testing AF-contaminated peanuts in the Philippines and back home,[36–39] I became aware of two phenomena: a seeming association between young Filipino children suffering from liver cancer and the consumption of animal protein, and the research results of a group in India testing the relationships among AF, liver cancer, and animal protein. Through this unlikely combination of circumstances, I came to see evidence of a surprising role for animal protein in developing liver cancer. I particularly wondered whether cancer growth initiated by AF might be accelerated by animal protein. Of course, this raised a serious issue for our project in the Philippines, and it put me in a difficult position. I could either continue advocating for the same high protein consumption and put these nagging questions out of my mind, or I could let them take me where they may, even if they led nowhere.

I think all of my work these past sixty-five-plus years clearly indicates which path I chose, why, and where it led me. Nagging questions almost always lead to more nagging questions, and when it comes to one's own biases, it's even more important that these questions are asked. So, what did I discover?

In the lab, I discovered that animal protein (but not plant protein) dramatically increased experimental cancer growth, and I uncovered evidence of at least ten biological mechanisms by which this animal protein effect could be explained, both in the early initiation phase of cancer and the later pro-motion phase. In parallel, I also discovered a wide range of international cor-relation studies that show a linear correlation of animal protein (or surrogate nutrients like saturated fat, which are most frequently packaged with ani-mal protein) with multiple cancers, cardiovascular disease, and other chronic diseases. Further, I found corroborating evidence from human intervention studies that have demonstrated the reversal of heart disease, diabetes, and other diseases with a diet free of animal-protein-based foods.

Some of this body of evidence challenges long-cherished beliefs of what good science and evidence looks like, and I will discuss those challenges at much greater length in Part III. The primary point I would like to make here is this: at some point in my career, whether by naïveté, clumsiness, or some other defect, I unwittingly undermined the most sacred, tacit agreement that binds together virtually all researchers in the field of nutrition—our centuries-old veneration of animal protein. The community's response to my conclusions testifies to the indelible imprint of animal protein on our collec-tive imagination.

As I described, one colleague explained to me that I had "fundamentally betrayed" the interests of the nutrition research community. Another, Profes-sor Alf Harper, who had written a very generous reference letter for my first professorship at Virginia Tech (while we were both at MIT), scolded me in a personal letter, in which he wrote that I had "fallen on my own petard." And perhaps there was some truth to that allegation, for sometimes I have noticed a strange sidelong glance from my peers, or some fear in their eyes, as if I am missing some crucial extremity that only they know about.

ERASED PREDECESSORS

You might wonder why there haven't been more critiques of the immoderate recommendations set by Voit and his contemporaries, which established the pattern of overconsumption that persists today. Surely, I am not the only one. As it turns out, certain outliers in the scientific community *did* question that early dogma. They have only been forgotten—or erased from the sanctioned history.

One such outlier was Russell Chittenden (1856–1943), a Yale professor and member of the US National Academy of Sciences. In his first of two prominent books on nutrition,[6,40] he cites the findings of several colleagues who had reported that low levels of protein (20–40 g/day) were sufficient for good health (remember, Voit and his colleagues advocated for 100–134 g/day).[6] But not only did Chittenden suggest a low-protein diet *could* work, he actually advocated for low-protein diets as a way to *improve* health. (Because "protein" generally meant animal-based protein at that time, when researchers like Chittenden say "low protein," they usually mean very little animal-based protein.)

In an experiment involving Yale freshmen in the Reserve Officer Training Corps program, Chittenden conducted a set of fifteen physical strength and endurance tests both before and after several months on a diet of less than 50 grams per day of protein (mostly plant-based). Their results, including averages, are included in the chart below. As you can see, the students did not wilt away as a result of their low-protein diets. Instead, each and every one showed significant improvement in their scores.

Name	October	April
Broyles	2560	5530
Coffman	2835	6269
Cohn	2210	4002
Fritz	2504	5178
Henderson	2970	4598
Loewenthal	2463	5277
Morris	2543	4869
Oakman	3445	5055
Silney	3245	5307
Steltz	2838	4581
Zooman	3070	5457
	2790	**5102**

In a second study, Chittenden enrolled already-fit athletes, who began with an average score of 4915, close to the final score of the first group.

Almost anyone who has ever exercised knows that the most significant gains often occur toward the beginning of a training regime, but on Chittenden's diet of low animal protein, even experienced athletes saw significant improvement in their scores.

Name	January	June
G. Anderson	4913	5722
W. Anderson	6016	9472
Bellis	5993	8165
Callahan	2154	3983
Donahue	4584	5917
Jacobus	4548	5667
Schenker	5728	7135
Stapleton	5351	6833
	4910	**6612**

If these results come as a surprise to you, you're not alone. It has long, wrongfully been assumed that athletic performance and recovery require a high-protein diet, a myth that persists even today. What Chittenden's experiments suggest (and did so more than a century ago!) is just the opposite. High performance does not require a high-protein diet. On the contrary, a low-protein diet can improve performance, regardless of baseline fitness.

As you might expect, though, Chittenden's findings were critiqued by some of his colleagues. The most common critique suggested that his subjects would have done even better on a high-protein diet. To test that hypothesis, you would also have to test physical performance in a group consuming a high-protein diet and compare their results.

Thankfully, such a test was conducted by another Yale professor, Irvine Fisher.[41] In his study, he compared "athletes accustomed to a high-protein and full-flesh dietary [with] athletes accustomed to a low-protein and non-flesh dietary." In addition to these two groups of athletes, he added a third group: "sedentary persons accustomed to a low-protein and non-flesh dietary." In the group of flesh-abstainers (i.e., those eating a plant-based diet), none of the subjects had eaten meat in the last two years, and most had adhered to that diet from four to twenty years. So, how did they do? Impressively, the first endurance test showed "great superiority on the side of the flesh-abstainers. Even the *maximum* record of the flesh-eaters was barely more than half the *average* for the flesh-abstainers." In two more tests, the flesh-abstainers again performed at a higher level.

What's particularly interesting, though, is that even the sedentary flesh-abstainers—couch potatoes whose diets consisted primarily of foods like, well, potatoes—outperformed the flesh-eating athletes. Concerned that there may have been more at play than strength and endurance alone—perhaps, the author speculates, the flesh-abstainers were more committed to proving their theory—"special pains were taken to stimulate the flesh-eaters to the utmost." Fisher describes one case in which "a Yale long distance runner" competed side by side with a "professor who had adopted the Chittenden diet." Despite (or perhaps because of?) his high-protein diet, the long-distance runner could not measure up to the professor in a challenge to see who could hold their arms outstretched for the longest: "in the course of a few minutes his arms began to tremble, and at the end of 8 minutes and 54 seconds they had gradually fallen . . . much to his mortification." Meanwhile, the professor maintained the pose for an additional *thirty-seven* minutes.*

---

* Chart key: Bat. Cr. = medical and other staff at Battle Creek Sanitarium; Yale = Yale students and instructors.

FIRST ENDURANCE TEST: HOLDING ARMS HORIZONTALLY

FLESH-EATERS ATHLETES‡		FLESH-ABSTAINERS†			
		ATHLETES‡		SEDENTARY	
NAMES	TIME IN MINUTES	NAMES	TIME IN MINUTES	NAMES	TIME IN MINUTES
L. B. Yale	6**	H. Bat. Or.	6	J. T. C. Bat. Or.	10
F. O. "	7**	N. "	6	E. L. E. "	10
C. H. C. "	7	A. B. "	10*	E. H. R. "	15
R. M. B. "	7	J. "	10	A. J. R. "	17
R. Ba. "	7	J. P. H. "	12	S. E. B. "	27
G. "	8	B. S. S. "	13	†I. F. Yale	37
F. S. N. "	8	S. "	13	P. R. Bat. Or.	42
W. J. H. "	9*	H. O. "	18*	J. F. M. "	51**
E. J. C. "	10	†W. B. B. Yale	16**	H. G. W. "	80
J. H. D. "	10	C. H. Bat. Or.	17	O. E. S. "	80
R. Bu. "	10	R. M. M. "	18	J. E. G. "	98*
H. A. R. "	12	O. A. "	21	A. W. N. "	170
C. S. M. "	14*	S. A. O. "	32	E. J. W. "	200
R. "	18	M. "	35		
G. K. "	22*	D. "	37		
		W. W. Yale	63		
		W. Bat Or.	75		
		†G. S. D. Yale	160		
		C. C. R. Bat. Or.	176*		
Average	**10**		**39**		**64**

*Limit of endurance. **Nearly to limit. †Fisher's indication of abstainers who occasionally ate flesh. ‡Defines "athletes" as either those in training for sports (among flesh-eaters) and those who trained for personal reasons (among abstainers).

More than a century has passed since Chittenden's and Fisher's landmark studies on the low-protein diet and its effects on athletic performance. In that time, there have been many other examples of modern athletes excelling after changing their diets to consume more whole plant foods and fewer animal foods. In 2005, the great golfer Gary Player asked my permission to speak about *The China Study* on the Golf Channel, one month after the book's publication. On bent knee, he implored all of America to read the book. At about the same time, Chris Campbell, the oldest-ever wrestler to win an Olympic medal and a Cornell law school graduate, invited me to speak to the US Olympic boxing team that he was coaching. Campbell himself was a vegan athlete. At the beginning of the 2007 NFL season, the greatest tight end of all time, Tony Gonzalez of the Kansas City Chiefs, phoned to say that he had read the book, changed his diet, and experienced the benefits. This in the lead-up to his eleventh season! Despite pressure from the team's and league's official nutritionist,* Gonzalez continued with great success. In early 2019, he was inducted into the Pro Football Hall of Fame. After a record fourteen Pro Bowl appearances, an unusually long seventeen-year career, and several all-time records, there's no doubt in my mind that his whole food, plant-based (WFPB) diet was more than sufficient to sustain his consistent world-class performance.

In the time since these icons reached out to me, I've been encouraged by more world-class athletes who have embraced a WFPB lifestyle and seen impressive improvements in their performance. This includes both endurance and power athletes, in as many sports as you can think of, across the globe. Even while working on this book, I learned that one-third of the Tennessee Titans NFL team has adopted a plant-based diet.[42] Last, more than a century after the groundbreaking work of Chittenden and Fisher, a documentary concerned with these very same questions, *Game Changers*, has been released. Proof, I think, that the public (and especially the public most concerned with achieving high performance, like athletes) is far more adaptable and forward thinking than the institutions that have strangled this discourse.†

But the remarkable fact remains that even with all this evidence of impressive athletic feats on a plant-based diet today, almost no one in the nutrition science profession has heard of Chittenden or Fisher's work. Whenever I mention this research, the response is always one of incredulity. Even among Yale alumni, Chittenden is a forgotten figure. The preeminent

---

* This nutritionist also held a leadership position in the Academy of Nutrition and Dietetics, the most prominent and influential dietetics society, which partners with the dairy, pharmaceutical, and soft drink industries.

† Another particularly promising development combining physical conditioning and the WFPB diet is the impressive strength and fitness training program founded by professional sports team consultant Jon Hinds. He now operates many gymnasiums around the US.[43] This fitness program and its gymnasia are advertised as "the only gyms in the nation to integrate full body skills training for strength, speed and stamina and a plant-based diet for the health of the planet." I receive no personal compensation from this organization and neither was I requested to make this comment.

Dr. Benjamin Spock, one of the bestselling and most influential authors of all time, whose book *The Common Sense Book of Baby and Child Care* has sold more than fifty million copies, once wrote to ask me about Chittenden after reading a commentary I had written for our newsletter.[44] Even as a Yale student during the early 1920s, an Olympic gold medalist as a member of the Yale crew, and a one-time vegetarian himself, Spock had never heard of Chittenden. He was puzzled why his coach had never told him and his fellow crew members of Chittenden's research, right there on the same campus. Instead, he was always told to eat lots of protein, and so gave up the vegetarian diet on which he had been raised. Much later in life, after learning of the macrobiotic diet and reading my comments on Chittenden, he reestablished his vegetarian diet.

Chittenden continued working, largely unnoticed, until he passed in 1943, the same year American Cancer Society founder Frederick Hoffman (see chapter two) passed. Although these men took two very different paths, they ultimately reached the same place. Both died as professional pariahs, hidden from public view. In another painful twist of fate, 1943 was also the first year that the United States Department of Agriculture, along with the National Academy of Medicine, made formal nutrient recommendations—recommendations that flew in the face of both men's research.

Over the next seventy-five years, programs following the USDA's 1943 nutrient recommendations have included the "Basic 7" food groups, the "Basic Four," the "Food Guide Pyramid," "MyPlate," and "MyPyramid," and are now called the US Dietary Guidelines. These various programs reflect a consistent paternalistic effort on the part of our government to maintain eating habits ordained as "healthy." By periodically freshening up their imaging and language, they have been able to mislead consumers into thinking that progress is being achieved. Despite these minor differences, however, there has been no progress beyond the view on protein forwarded by Voit and his colleagues so long ago. Today's guidelines continue to allow and even encourage excessive consumption of protein, in particular "high-quality" animal-based protein, and as long as that remains the case, any "progress" in their recommendations will remain superficial and insufficient.

I'll say it again: it's remarkable that almost no one has heard of Chittenden. The same is true of Hoffman. But is it surprising? They shared many characteristics—including being treated like ghosts before their deaths—so why not this erasure from history, too? In the work of both men, the benefits of the low-protein diet were clear, or at least highly provocative and worthy of further research. And in both cases, that work was ignored.

GROUPTHINK: THE INVISIBLE FENCE

We have seen by now how our cultural beliefs about animal protein have biased us away from certain individuals and their research, past and present, and toward other kinds of research, methods, recommendations, and assumptions. The resistance against unorthodox views is often flagrant, measured in professional careers lost, huge numbers of actual lives prematurely lost, and money wasted. But it also often goes unrecognized.

This is precisely why I call our collective reverence of animal protein a cult: because that reverence, and its consequences, so often goes unrecognized. Innocent obliviousness, a hallmark of cult members, is the best explanation for why more well-intentioned people don't protest the animal protein status quo. Within cults, the flow of information is often significantly restricted, resulting in "groupthink." This is something I've seen and experienced many times, both within the field of nutrition, and more broadly. A popular term in psychology, groupthink is a spin-off and extension of the experimental lingo that appears in George Orwell's *Nineteen Eighty-Four*. It was originally studied in 1972 by Yale research psychologist Irving Janis,[45,46] but there's since been much more research on this concept. As a starting point, I rather like the definition provided by Wikipedia:

> *A psychological phenomenon that occurs within a group of people in which the desire for harmony or conformity in the group results in an irrational or dysfunctional decision-making outcome. Group members try to minimize conflict and reach a consensus decision without critical evaluation of alternative viewpoints by actively suppressing dissenting viewpoints, and by isolating themselves from outside influences.*[45]

But groupthink is more than just the *consequence* of restricted information; it also *causes* further restriction of information. In other words, it operates as a positive feedback loop: the more homogenous our thinking, the more likely we are to restrict the flow of alternative information, which in turn produces even more homogenization, and so on and so forth, until the group in question is absolutely paralyzed by its inescapable tendency to conform.

Unsurprisingly, groupthink has had an "extensive reach . . . in the field of communications studies, political science, management, and organizational theory."[43] Perhaps the most common example of the phenomenon is when organizations get caught up in a scandal: even those not directly implicated look the other way, and misconduct is "covered up in the hopes of saving the institution's reputation, and the money that accompanies it." The reason this happens is because institutions "inspire emotion. They inspire loyalty. And they have established ways of doing things that rev up when problems surface . . . most relevantly, they often have a community built around them, geographically or otherwise."[47]

Sometimes, though, scandal involves no cover-up. Indeed, the greatest scandals often sit in plain sight. This is how groupthink at its most insidious operates, more often than not, in the field of nutrition. It is by this process that the field of nutrition has abjectly refused to acknowledge challenges against animal protein. Researchers in the field are merely defending the premise that maintains their authority, and doing so by whatever means possible. If a group has been tethered from the very start to a reverence for animal protein, then why should we expect the group to admit opposing evidence?

Many of us understand groupthink intimately. Perhaps you can remember a situation from your own life in which you discovered something that didn't quite jibe with the status quo. Perhaps you even spoke out and disrupted the harmony of a group you once belonged to. I know it can be a very difficult task. We are often unaware of groupthink's control over us. It's easy to see the fault in another group, but not so easy in our own. Assuming we could even spot all the limiting parameters that govern our groups, the repercussions of speaking out are often serious and unavoidable. Who among us wants to be shunned or labeled a crank? And so, it is groupthink that swallows individual thought. It's happened many times before: to you, to me, to critics of the local theory of cancer, to Chittenden and Fisher and countless others whose names no longer register as important, if they ever did. As long as humanity exists, I'm sure groupthink will continue to affect many areas of life, often without any fanfare or hullabaloo, but instead rather like the wind—not seen but only felt.

In a small number of groupthink cases, there may be some bad actors, but I believe these are rare. More likely, people with the power to change simply think they know better; they do not realize what damaging myths lurk in their blind spots. They have grown comfortable in confinement and find others' freedom threatening. Such is the outsized sensitivity surrounding animal protein that they will even struggle against the dissemination of information that could save lives.

A few years ago, the success of our nonprofit's online plant-based nutrition certificate course came to the attention of the communications office at Cornell, which publishes *The Cornell Chronicle*, a university bullhorn for alumni that celebrates notable achievements on campus. I've long found the communications office to be very helpful, and in fact, they publicized our research program for more than forty years. I was told in the late nineties by a retired writer for that office that our work was the most publicized of any being done at Cornell during that forty-year period, in line with that of a colleague, the famous astronomer Carl Sagan. In any case, about five years ago one of their senior writers proposed a news release on the unusual successes of our online plant-based nutrition course (which had the highest enrollment of any on eCornell). As a part of that news release, the writer wanted to include a few testimonials of celebrities who had recommended our book *The China Study*, as well as the president of Cornell himself, David Skorton, MD, who was a vegetarian. Unfortunately, Skorton first sought the advice of his advisers. I'm confident it was pressure from the director of the Division of Nutritional Sciences and the deans of the College of Agriculture and Life Sciences and the College of Human Ecology that caused him to absent himself from the news release, and to kill the story in *The Cornell Chronicle*.

The public demand for our course was, understand, *controversial* news.

Technically *The Cornell Chronicle* is owned by the university and, as such, the university has the legal authority to unilaterally control all of its content (as I was advised by attorney Floyd Abrams, a Cornell alum and the most famous American scholar of the First Amendment).[48,49] Fair enough from a legal perspective, but where does that leave the public? How are they to learn about our professionally published research findings of some forty years?

As long as reputable, public-facing institutions like Cornell University exercise their legally protected silence, where will the public learn of new research advances obtained there? Are those findings to be sequestered in professional research journals mostly inaccessible to the public? When there comes a conflict between the university's interests and the public's interest, will the public ever win out?

Until recently, most academic research studies have been *funded by the American taxpayer* (in more recent times, much of that share of funding has shifted to the private sector). Once this public-funded research is completed, the scientific reliability of its findings are then carefully judged by scientifically qualified peers before being deemed worthy of publication in professional journals. But unfortunately, given the costliness of subscription, most of the public will never have access to those publications, and even if they did, thanks to the impenetrable jargon used in most scientific writing, most would struggle to understand the findings. Laypeople have to rely entirely on professional interpretation of research studies, or else never receive the information they have paid for. And the rationale behind the kind of information control that occurred here, in respect to the innocuous news of our online course's success, raises serious red flags. What additional information do Cornell administrators have that supersedes that of professional scientists, particularly in the case of publicly funded research?

Freedom of speech is an incredibly important right. I suspect James Madison knew what he was doing when he put it first! But when freedom of speech swallows the individual journalist's agency, when it muzzles the individual researcher's findings, and when it shortchanges the public taxpayer—serious questions must be asked of *the speaker*.

The following pictures are from a relatively new Cornell building dedicated to dairy science. (Ironically, the older version of this fine building once housed my graduate student office.) They attest to that old adage that a picture is worth a thousand words. In this case, however, I worry they're worth more than just words. Painfully for me, they illustrate what Cornell values more: not free speech, but the contributions and input of industry.

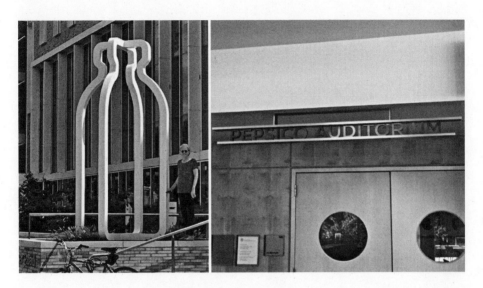

And so, how can we trust Cornell and other powerful academic institutions to mediate fairly when publicly funded research threatens industry? Even more doubtful—how can we trust them in the case of highly privileged and prioritized industries, such as those entrusted with promoting and profiting from the sacred cow of all nutrition, animal protein?

CHAPTER SIX

RELATED MYTHS, DEBATES, AND DIVERSIONS

*The good and evil resulting from our words and
deeds go on apportioning themselves.*
—José Saramago

I have given special attention to animal protein, and our continued attachment to it, in this part of the book not because there are no other points of confusion and misunderstanding in nutrition, but because protein, and animal protein in particular, has long been a treasured nutrient. It is what I call a "driver nutrient": our valuation of it determines, more than any other nutrient, our dietary choices and public policy positions. All discussions on the meaning of nutrition have been distorted by our valuation of animal protein. And I do not believe that its high valuation is warranted by acceptable science, but rather comes from a long history of fallacy.

The primary consequences of our outsized emphasis on animal protein consumption are elaborated in chapter five (misleading measures of protein quality, misguided policy efforts both at home and abroad, and a refusal to acknowledge contradictory research). But I'm equally disturbed by its secondary effects. Our attachment to animal protein, as a driver nutrient, has triggered numerous misconceptions not mentioned in chapter five. It has had a profound effect on our understanding of other nutrients and practices, and I want to discuss a few of these knock-on effects here.

#1: DIETARY CHOLESTEROL

Most people believe that the cholesterol we consume (dietary cholesterol) is responsible for the levels of cholesterol in our blood (serum cholesterol). By extension, most believe that dietary cholesterol is the single most important cause of heart disease. These ideas have persisted for a century. The public continues to imagine that heart attacks are caused by blood vessels clogged up with cholesterol; policy makers have recommended maximum levels of cholesterol intake; and attempts have been made to breed animals with lower levels of cholesterol in their meat or edible products.[1] Our preoccupation with cholesterol is clear. The food and pharmaceutical industries have been more than happy to encourage this belief, investing hundreds of billions of dollars—surely more than a trillion when adjusted for inflation—in the research and development of products designed to minimize the harm caused by cholesterol. This includes both the marketing of cholesterol-lowering foods and the creation and marketing of cholesterol-lowering medications. As for the scientific community, more than 270,000 publications on the Library of Medicine's PubMed website refer to cholesterol.

However, some of the most interesting research on this subject was conducted during the early 1900s. Using laboratory animals, these century-old studies showed that animal-based foods such as meat, milk, and eggs caused early signs of heart disease and higher blood cholesterol.[2,3] During the next ten to fifteen years, at least ten different research groups attempted to identify the factor in these animal foods that might explain these effects.[4,5] Dietary cholesterol, they hypothesized, might be one such factor, because it is only found in animal foods. However, during the 1920s,[6-8] these experimental animal studies in effect collectively concluded that *animal protein* was more responsible for increased blood cholesterol than dietary cholesterol itself. As one report said, in reflecting on these earlier studies, "elevation of blood cholesterol . . . [is] directly referable to the excess of protein in the diet and not to its cholesterol content."[9] These experimental findings suggested that a diet low in cholesterol but high in animal protein would increase blood cholesterol more than a diet low in animal protein. Several decades later, Ancel Keys, who was and remains one of the most quoted and influential of all heart disease researchers, also suggested that "it is now clear that dietary cholesterol, per se . . . has little to no effect on the serum cholesterol concentration in man."[10,11] If this sounds surprising to you, you're not alone. As established above, many in the public still believe that the cholesterol we consume directly increases blood cholesterol and its partner, cardiovascular disease.

From 1940 to 1990, even more evidence emerged from both experimental animal studies and human studies suggesting that animal-based protein is the major cause of heart disease, certainly more so than plant-based protein or dietary cholesterol.[12-21] Perhaps the most convincing evidence on the effects of animal protein on heart disease was presented in a book of nine manuscripts published in 1983.[22] In the first of those manuscripts, the authors review early research efforts and conclude that "the contribution of protein to the development and progression of atherosclerosis is gaining new recognition . . . building on the observation made over 70 years ago." Sadly, nothing ever materialized from this "new recognition" in the early 1980s. These papers were mostly ignored by the nutrition science community and never reached the public.

And what about plant protein? Does a similar connection exist between plant protein and serum cholesterol? The answer is no, and the experimental research published from 1940 to 1990 is most convincing, especially the research on soy protein. In 1941, soy protein was shown to decrease early atherosclerosis in experimental animals by 70 to 80 percent compared to casein, the chief protein in cow's milk.[23,24] Lactalbumin, another cow's milk protein, also increased serum cholesterol, triglycerides, and atherosclerosis compared to soy protein.[18,25] Even in short-term studies, switching proteins produced a dramatic effect. When the protein in the animals' diets was switched from casein to soy protein, lowered blood cholesterol appeared within a single day, whereas switching from soy to casein increased blood cholesterol within twenty-four hours—an effect lasting at least twenty days.[21,26] My lab's research a few years later showed a similar rapid effect: diets high in casein (20 percent of total calories) stimulated cancer growth quickly, and diets low in casein quickly reversed that growth. Last, although low-fat diets decrease blood cholesterol in human studies, that decrease is minimal compared to the tenfold greater effect of replacing animal protein with soy protein.[27,28]

The size of soy protein's reducing effect seemed unusually promising. You would think it might have sparked debates about plant versus animal foods, raised questions about the dietary cholesterol theory, or driven discussion about the greater context of nutrition in general. Unfortunately, this wasn't the case. Many researchers interpreted the soy protein effect as a specific effect of soy rather than a possible broader effect of plant foods.[14] This was likely because, at the time, the blood cholesterol levels and incidence of atherosclerosis associated with animal-protein diets (though not *because of* animal protein, per se) were already considered a normal biological response. If one mindlessly accepts animal protein diets as normal, soy protein and its effects seem like an anomaly. But what if the opposite were true? What if the much-lower blood cholesterol levels and atherosclerosis incidence associated with soy protein (and plant food consumption generally) are Nature's true norm? Rather than framing soy protein as unusually protective, what if we had considered animal protein as usually damaging?

Instead of pursuing that line of thought, researchers did not question the normalcy of animal protein and its punishing effects on human health. Meanwhile, industry did what industry does best. Big Soy leveraged these findings on soy protein and cholesterol to gain a foothold in a market long dominated by animal foods. Between 1970 and 2000, the underdog soy and the behemoth dairy industries jockeyed for consumers' attention, each relying on their own set of health claims and leaving the public increasingly confused. Granted, the health claims advertised by the soy industry were more scientifically valid, but the point remains that neither industry encouraged the public to think about the broader context of plant and animal foods.

It's hardly surprising that the soy industry—as well as the other plant-based milks and other food products that have emerged to compete both alongside and against soy since the early 2000s—took this shortcut to profit. What's more disturbing is the scientific community's continued deference to the dietary cholesterol theory. For too long we have been willing to accept the idea that dietary cholesterol causes atherosclerosis, despite many contradictory findings. I believe this is because the alternative would require an about-face on the entire history of nutrition. As outlined in chapter five, animal protein had already been celebrated as the greatest of all nutrients for several decades by the early twentieth century, when research questioning its role in disease emerged, only to be quickly ignored. The early twentieth century was also when new analytical methods emerged for measuring so-called biological value,[29] methods that invariably favored the consumption of animal foods.

As for the public, I believe many accept the theory about dietary cholesterol not only because they don't know any better, but also because it allows for the continued consumption of animal foods. (I'm reminded of my friend Dick Warner, discussed in chapter four, who was happy to eat low-fat foods but had a more difficult time giving up meat.) Whereas cholesterol and saturated fat can easily be removed from animal foods, as in the case of skim milk and lean cuts of meat, the removal of protein would result in a far less appetizing dinner party. Once you remove the protein from cow's milk, for example, you are left with an inedible emulsion of fat, water, and a touch of milk sugar. Imagine drinking such a smoothie!

Eventually, the nutrition research community's focus shifted somewhat gradually away from dietary cholesterol and toward fat, especially saturated fat. In fact, this increased focus on saturated fat is a part of my own life. In the mid-1940s, I woke every morning before dawn to milk two cows by hand for our consumption on the family farm (until my dad decided to enlarge our herd, at which point we introduced milking machines). In those days, heifers were valued by the pedigrees of their parents (dam and sire), by the amount of milk they produced, and by that milk's butterfat content. In the late '40s, however, my dad began to hear that high-fat milk might not be as precious as commonly believed. Thereafter, once we set aside some of the milk for our personal use, we began centrifuging out the fat from the rest to make butter, again mostly for our own use, then feeding the remaining skim milk to the pigs. I still remember the tedium of centrifuging the milk with a hand-turned machine.

Looking back on those days, knowing what I now know, I'm confident that the messages coming down to farmers like my dad likely arose from the early writings of Ancel Keys. In 1952, he suggested that "nutritional evidence points to a small need for dietary fats as such" and that the then-existing recommendation of 30 to 40 percent fat in one's diet "could be lowered . . . to 15 to 25 percent of total calories . . . without any nutritional harm."[30] Somewhat later, Keys began his famous Seven Countries Study in the Mediterranean countries and Japan, which supported his theory that saturated fat, rather than cholesterol, was most to blame for high levels of cholesterol in our blood.[31,32] Although his conclusions about saturated fat are flawed given what we know today (I will discuss saturated fat shortly), his critique of the widely held beliefs about cholesterol remains valid.

Nevertheless, many continued to chiefly blame dietary cholesterol for high levels of blood cholesterol and related diseases such as atherosclerosis, largely encouraged by the authoritative food and health policy "experts" who, until the 2002 edition of the dietary guidelines, set intake recommendations for cholesterol.[33] By emphasizing the role of dietary cholesterol in disease formation, we have unwittingly sacrificed millions of lives. We have preserved animal protein as a nutrient of prime importance; created an entirely new, phony market for "healthy" meats and dairy; and laid the groundwork for the commercial development of cholesterol-lowering drugs like statins and procedures like stents, all the while promoting the false impression that our scientific understanding is evolving.

#2: SATURATED FAT: A SCAPEGOAT AND DISTRACTION FROM ANIMAL PROTEIN

When it became known that saturated fat consumption was associated with higher levels of blood cholesterol and heart disease,[10,34,35] thanks to the work of the aforementioned Ancel Keys, saturated fats were quickly labeled "bad fats." Conversely, unsaturated fats, which were associated with lower levels of blood cholesterol and less heart disease, were labeled "good fats." Unfortunately, this exceptionally simplistic distinction has largely missed the point, resulting in a great deal of unnecessary confusion.

Before addressing why, I would like to briefly explain what each of these terms mean. I hope you will forgive me for dipping my toes into some molecular-level detail, but I think it may help to draw a more complete picture. In the chart, you can see the three primary categories of fat: saturated, unsaturated, and trans. Unsaturated fat, in turn, can be further subdivided into monounsaturated and polyunsaturated fat.

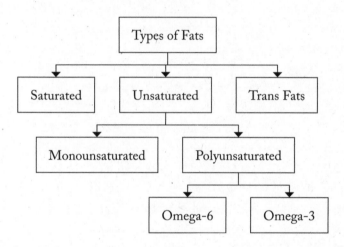

The most basic difference between saturated fat, or saturated fatty acids, and unsaturated fat, or unsaturated fatty acids, is that saturated fat is solid at room temperature and generally associated with animal foods (e.g., butter, lard), and unsaturated fat is liquid at room temperature and generally associated with plant foods (e.g., corn oil, olive oil). But on a molecular level, the difference between them has to do with their chemical structures. All fatty acids, saturated or unsaturated, are made up of a chain of carbon atoms. At one end of this carbon chain is the acid end, $-COOH$, and at the other, the methyl end, CH_3-. Fatty acids are further distinguished by the length of their carbon (C) chain and by the type of chemical bond linking these carbon atoms together. Most fatty acids have an even number of carbon atoms, though some have an odd number, and they are often described as short chain (2–6 carbons), medium chain (8–12 carbons), or long chain (14–24 carbons). If every C in the chain is linked with two hydrogen (H) atoms, the fatty acid is said to be *saturated*. Conversely, if there is only one H atom for one or more pairs of carbon neighbors, it is considered *unsaturated* (–CH=CH–). If, in the entire fatty acid chain, there is only one unsaturated bond, it is *monounsaturated* (e.g., olive oil); if there is more than one, it is *polyunsaturated* (e.g., corn oil).

$$H-\underset{\underset{H}{|}}{\overset{\overset{H}{|}}{C}}-\underset{\underset{H}{|}}{\overset{\overset{H}{|}}{C}}-\underset{\underset{H}{|}}{\overset{\overset{H}{|}}{C}}-\underset{\underset{H}{|}}{\overset{\overset{H}{|}}{C}}-\underset{\underset{H}{|}}{\overset{\overset{H}{|}}{C}}-\overset{\overset{O}{\|}}{C}-OH$$

Saturated Fatty Acid

$$H-\underset{\underset{H}{|}}{\overset{\overset{H}{|}}{C}}-\underset{\underset{H}{|}}{\overset{\overset{H}{|}}{C}}-\overset{\overset{H}{|}}{C}=\overset{\overset{H}{|}}{C}-\underset{\underset{H}{|}}{\overset{\overset{H}{|}}{C}}-\overset{\overset{O}{\|}}{C}-OH$$

Monounsaturated Fatty Acid

$$H-\overset{\overset{H}{|}}{C}=\overset{\overset{H}{|}}{C}=\overset{\overset{H}{|}}{C}=\overset{\overset{H}{|}}{C}=\overset{\overset{H}{|}}{C}-\overset{\overset{O}{\|}}{C}-OH$$

Polyunsaturated Fatty Acid

Additionally, fatty acids are commonly linked to a glycerol molecule, which may bind one, two, or three fatty acids together, thus becoming a mono-, di-, or triglyceride. In the following triglyceride model, each fatty acid is a chain of ten carbon atoms, the top two chains saturated and the bottom chain monounsaturated.

■ Glycerol ■ Carboxyl Group ■ Fatty Acid = Double Bond

Now, as I have already said, when it comes to the foods we eat, *saturated fats are generally associated with animal foods* and *unsaturated fats are generally associated with plant foods*. Still, this distinction is somewhat simplistic. In point of fact, it would be more accurate to say that animal foods have a higher *proportion* of saturated fat, and that plant foods have a higher *proportion* of unsaturated fat. The proportions of saturated, monounsaturated, and polyunsaturated fatty acids in various foods and food fats are shown in the following chart.

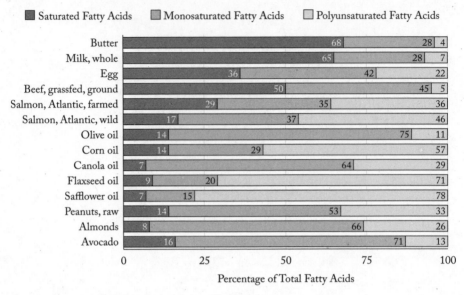

Source: Oregon State University, Linus Pauling Institute.

Now, given how nuanced the differences are between these fatty acids on a molecular level, why is it that we so often hear unsaturated fat simplistically described as "good fat" and saturated fat simplistically described as "bad fat"? The origin of these labels is illustrated in the following three charts, which show associations for a large-scale, international correlation study that became highly influential in the professional community, and generally among the public.[36] The first chart shows a direct relationship between *total dietary fat* intake and age-adjusted death rates for breast cancer (total fat includes both saturated and unsaturated fat). This association has had a major influence on food and health policy recommendations for decades.[37–42] However, the straight-line association of disease death rates for total fat (the first chart) is much better explained as an effect of saturated fat specifically (the second chart), as no such association exists for unsaturated fat (the third chart).

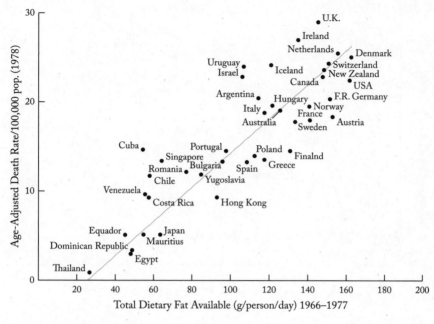

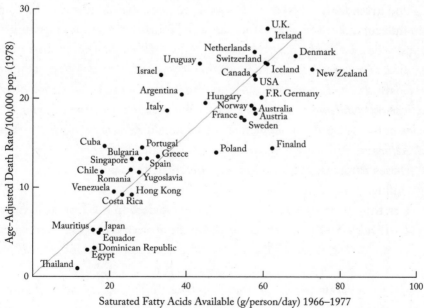

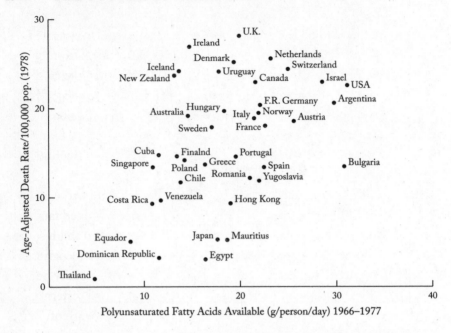

Understandably, when these associations were first discovered, the common interpretation was that saturated fat was "bad fat" and that unsaturated fat was "good fat," or at the very least harmless fat. And although this interpretation may *feel* satisfying, I believe that it is deeply flawed. Here I come to the most important point of this section: *I propose that the impressive disease association of total and saturated fat would be much better interpreted as an association of disease with animal protein, which just happens to be highly correlated with saturated fat.*[43]

There is more evidence to support this interpretation:

1. In a cohort of nearly 90,000 women studied in the Harvard Nurses' Health Study, breast cancer risk did not decrease as expected when dietary fat declined from 50 to 55 percent of total calories to 20 to 25 percent.[44,45] If anything, as the principal author has often pointed out, there was a slight *increase* in disease risk (though not statistically significant), possibly related to a higher concentration of protein in these low-fat diets.

2. Biochemically speaking, saturated fat is relatively inert. Thus, it is an unlikely cause of disease. If anything, unsaturated fat is

more likely to be the culprit in disease formation. Unsaturated fat is more biologically active, contributes to the formation of highly reactive oxygen species that promote diseases like cancer and heart disease, and promotes cancer more than saturated fat in experimental animal studies. For example, corn oil (rich in unsaturated fat) is considerably more cancer promoting than coconut oil,[46–48] which is an unusual plant oil in that it contains higher levels of saturated fat.

3. As a highly reputable group of Australian researchers wrote in 2014, "More than five decades have passed since saturated fats were first reported as a major cause of hypercholesterolemia [high serum cholesterol]. Saturated fats have consequently become recognized as a major etiological factor in the development of coronary heart disease and source of morbidity and mortality in the Western world . . . Despite this commonly held belief and a wealth of epidemiological and intervention studies over the last fifty years, conclusive evidence establishing a link between intake of saturated fatty acids and blood cholesterol levels does not exist . . . [and] the mechanism by which this [cause–effect association] would occur still remains unclear."[49] This point is critical: *There is no convincing empirical evidence showing how saturated fat causes or initiates disease formation, for either cancer or heart disease.*

4. As stated in an even more recent 2018 interview by one of the Australian authors, "There appears to be no consistent benefit to all-cause or cardiovascular disease mortality from the reduction of dietary saturated fat."[50]

5. Alternative explanations for the "fat effect" exist. For example, in a 1979 human intervention study, a low-fat diet decreased serum cholesterol minimally compared to a low-fat, soy protein diet.[27,51] In other words, removing animal protein had the more profound effect.

Despite the gaps in our understanding of how saturated fat could cause disease, it has been widely vilified for decades. Why? I propose that this has been a convenient alibi to avoid our blaming the real cause, animal-protein-based foods. As I just noted, saturated fat is not particularly chemically reactive, a property required for causing a disease or initiating events that promote a disease.

A great deal of confusion has been generated by the weak and questionable evidence supporting the hypothesis that total and saturated fat (along with cholesterol) are to blame for disease. Many devout meat consumers point out the very real flaws in this evidence in order to make the argument that saturated fat is not so bad (scientifically valid), but then leap to the conclusion that the animal foods often identified with saturated fat must also be not so bad (scientifically invalid). Although it is true that saturated fat is not the villain many believe it to be, it is still associated with disease. And the reason, too often ignored, is that saturated fat is *an excellent stand-in for animal protein*. By blaming *only* the surrogate, we are completely missing the greater context: that animal-protein-containing foods, such a huge part of most Western diets, are highly determinative of cancers and heart disease.

Unlike saturated fat, there are numerous biochemical mechanisms linking animal protein consumption to disease. Unlike saturated fat, animal protein is not biologically inert; on the contrary, increased consumption of animal protein has been proven to increase free radical oxidation, growth hormone activities, and more. And critically, unlike saturated fat, animal protein cannot be removed from animal foods.

#3: TRANS FATS, OMEGA-3S, AND OMEGA-6S

Just as saturated fats have been unfairly demonized as "bad fat," so too have unsaturated fats been inappropriately celebrated as "good fat." This falsehood is a direct consequence of our ignoring the damaging effects of animal protein consumption, which raises a whole new set of problems.

One such problem is trans fats. When it became evident that the consumption of unsaturated fats was associated with less cholesterol consumption and less heart disease, everyone wanted to replace the "bad" saturated fats of animal-based foods with these "good" fats of plant-based foods. But it is not easy to replace saturated fats with whole food sources of unsaturated fats. Chopped walnuts do not spread over toast as easily as butter. Neither do the so-called good oils extracted and isolated from plants (leaving aside for the moment that the benefits of unsaturated fats were seen only when eaten in *whole plant foods*, not in isolated oils). Eventually, the puzzle was solved: by bubbling hydrogen through the oil (with a catalyst) to saturate, at least partially, its double bonds with hydrogen atoms, plant oils could be solidified, allowing for them to be spread (e.g., oleomargarine, Crisco). "Good fats" thus became more versatile—they could be used either as liquids or solids, depending on one's preferences, and could even appease those who preferred the familiarity of butter.

There are issues with this artificial saturation, however. In it, hydrogen atoms do not line up as perfectly as in nature, and a small but significant number of hydrogen atoms attach to opposite sides of the fatty acid chain, creating what's known as a trans fat. To cut a long story short, it later became evident that trans fats significantly increase the risk of disease, especially heart disease, and regulatory agencies began making considerable efforts to keep them out of the marketplace.

This story illustrates both the seductiveness of technical solutions, which we so often pursue instead of paying attention to Nature's context, and the usual inadequacy of those solutions. We wanted to replace our "bad fats" with "good fats"—an understandable if faulty premise—but it wasn't logical to then chemically *transform* those "good fats" to make them more familiar or versatile. Besides, unsaturated fats are far more complicated than the early correlation studies suggested. We certainly should not embrace them all as healthy, without considering their context, especially the context of different levels of total fat.

One of the most important shifts in our investigations of unsaturated fats has been the focus on two of the best-known fatty acid types, omega-3 and omega-6 fats. One of my graduate students conducted further studies on the ability of these fats to modify experimental pancreatic cancer, the findings of which were published in and featured on the cover of the *Journal of the National Cancer Institute*.[52,53] In brief, they showed that omega-3 fats inhibited cancer growth while omega-6 fats promoted cancer growth; both results were consistent with later studies by others showing, respectively, these fats' anti- and pro-inflammatory properties.

This brings us to the question: How might we incorporate this information on omega fats into the conversation surrounding unsaturated fats?

Again, I think it may be useful to briefly describe some biochemical-level details. Omega-3 and omega-6 fatty acids (also known as n-3 and n-6, or alpha-linolenic acid, ALA, and linoleic acid, LA, respectively) are both essential to healthy body function, when in the correct balance. Our bodies cannot make either of them and so we must consume both. The designations omega-3 and omega-6 refer to the previously discussed placement of their double bonds in the fatty acid molecule, counting from the methyl (CH_3, at left in the chart below) end of the molecule.

Linoleic acid (18:2 n-6)
Omega-6 fatty acid with double bonds at positions 6 and 9 counting from the methyl group

α-Linoleic Acid (18:3 n-3)
Omega-3 fatty acid with double bonds at positions 3, 6, and 9 counting from the methyl group

Minor though it may seem, the position of the double bond makes a significant difference: omega-6 fatty acids are *pro-inflammatory* (capable of promoting chronic diseases like heart disease), while omega-3 fatty acids are *anti-inflammatory* (capable of inhibiting these diseases). Decades' worth of research show that these omega fats function through many mechanisms to produce a variety of health and disease outcomes. Unfortunately, though unsurprisingly, this popular distinction between anti-inflammatory omega-3s and pro-inflammatory omega-6s is too simplistic, and these nutrients are often discussed in conflicting and confusing ways—mostly because they are discussed as if they operate independently.

There are several reasons for the confusion surrounding omega-3 and omega-6 fatty acids. First and perhaps most critically, *these nutrients do not behave the same in whole foods as they do in supplements*. Despite a tremendous amount of marketing, the science is clear: they do not act independently (i.e., in supplement form) to support long-term health. One report, published in

2018, and "the most extensive systematic assessment of effects of n-3 fats on cardiovascular health to date ... concluded that omega-3 supplements do not work."[54] But omega-3 supplements—indeed, supplements generally—are an easy sell. Many consumers would like to believe in their value, as they are quite literally an easier pill to swallow than the kind of dietary change that produces real health. A second reason for the confusion surrounding omega-3 and omega-6 fatty acids is that the conversation often ignores qualifying conditions (e.g., varying amounts of other nutrients in the diet being tested) that influence these nutrients' function. And third, both omega-3 and omega-6 fatty acids are metabolized into distinct families of chemical products that support these fatty acids' anti- and pro-inflammatory functions, respectively, and it is not always clear which of these products (metabolites) are relevant because internal cellular conditions change constantly. All of these sources of confusion have something important in common: they each ignore biological context.

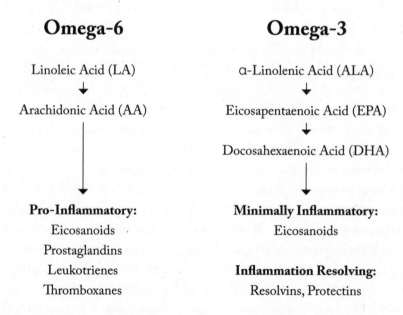

Omega-6	Omega-3
Linoleic Acid (LA)	α-Linolenic Acid (ALA)
↓	↓
Arachidonic Acid (AA)	Eicosapentaenoic Acid (EPA)
	↓
	Docosahexaenoic Acid (DHA)
↓	↓
Pro-Inflammatory:	**Minimally Inflammatory:**
Eicosanoids	Eicosanoids
Prostaglandins	
Leukotrienes	**Inflammation Resolving:**
Thromboxanes	Resolvins, Protectins

The balance of omega-3 and omega-6 fats within the body, *expressed as a ratio*, is far more important than the consumption of specific amounts of either fat in isolation—because, as previously said, it is the balance that matters most. I'm impressed by the research of Artemis Simopolous, MD, who persuasively argues for the importance of this balance or ratio.[55,56] The most obvious reason for reframing the omega-3–omega-6 discussion to focus on this ratio rather than these fatty acids' individual consumption is that it emphasizes the interdependence between them. It appreciates the fact that the effects observed from the nutrients we consume are the result of multiple mechanisms acting synergistically within the body—a unique departure from our conventional study of nutrition.

When we consider fat consumption from this perspective, the radical transformation of our diet during the twentieth century becomes apparent. Our omega-6:omega-3 ratio has increased from an evolutionary low point of 1:1 to today's 20:1 or even higher.[55] This illustrates a profound shift to the consumption of foods that contain more omega-6 and less omega-3. The biological consequences of such a shift are well documented, including increased "blood viscosity, vasospasm, and vasoconstriction" in heart disease and changes in many more mechanisms that contribute to diabetes, obesity, and cancer.[55]

How have we achieved such a pro-inflammatory diet? One explanation is the rise of industrial livestock production. To maximize growth and production on factory farms, animals have been fed increasingly large amounts of grain, especially corn, which is especially high in omega-6 fatty acids.[57] As a result, the concentration of omega-6s in the tissue of these animals is much higher than in the grass-fed cattle or wild game of yesteryear. This change is further exacerbated, of course, by the increase in the number of animal-based foods we eat. As industrial meat, dairy, and egg sources have become a larger part of our diets, so too have higher concentrations of omega-6 fatty acids. Said another way, our voracious consumption of "high-quality" animal protein has dramatically, dangerously skewed our omega-6:omega-3 ratio.

Another explanation for the increasing omega-6:omega-3 ratio has to do with the conversion of the parent omega-3 fatty acid (ALA) into its biologically active metabolites (EPA and DHA). The task of converting ALA into EPA, and converting EPA into DHA, requires the activity of a certain enzyme. However, evidence now suggests that omega-6 fatty acids compete for the same enzyme activity. This means that if the body already contains a high concentration of omega-6 fatty acids, the conversion of omega-3 fatty acids into their biologically active metabolites will be restricted, further exacerbating the problem.

The third and perhaps most significant explanation for this rising ratio is the increased consumption of added oils. As you can see in the chart below, except for flaxseed oil, most added oils contain large proportions of omega-6 fatty acids. These oils are susceptible to oxidation, cause inflammation, and are ubiquitous in our modern era of "convenience" foods. This is why poly-unsaturated fatty acids—*when consumed as added oil*—are not "good fat" and should not be viewed as such. You may recall this point from the saturated fat section above: unsaturated fats as added oils promote cancer and other chronic, degenerative diseases under experimental conditions more efficiently than do relatively inert saturated fats.[46-48] (Note that this chart also shows omega-9 fatty acids, which contain only one double bond.)

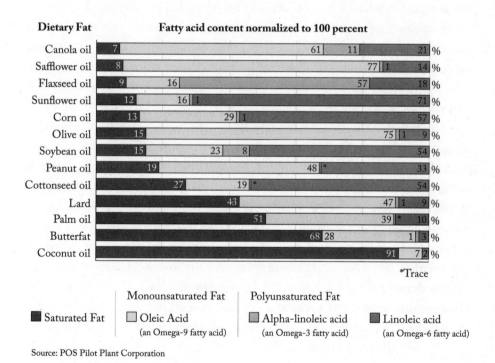

Source: POS Pilot Plant Corporation

The good news is that polyunsaturated fats in the context of whole foods behave differently than when they are extracted from plants and put into a bottle. Whole foods contain many antioxidative factors (antioxidants, minerals), and are thus able to control the damage of free radical production that otherwise might occur when these oils are consumed in isolation, such as added oils. Whereas the consumption of isolated oils should be avoided to minimize risk of heart disease, cancer, obesity, and related chronic diseases, whole plant foods containing these fats (nuts, seeds, avocados, etc.) are generally nutritious when consumed in moderation. For instance, according to a huge pooled analysis of fifteen studies on nut consumption (355,000 subjects, 3.8 million person-years), one serving of nuts per week and per day resulted in a 4 percent and 27 percent *lower* death rate for all-cause deaths, and a 7 percent and 39 percent *lower* death rate for cardiovascular diseases, respectively. Cancer death rate was *lower* by 14 percent.[58] A 2017 summary of fourteen studies showed that nut consumption was associated with lower risk of cardiovascular disease, lower risk of hypertension, and lower levels of total blood cholesterol.[59]

I realize that I have covered a significant amount of information in this and the previous section, including specific details pertaining to molecular composition and function. If some of these details still seem confusing to you, please don't be concerned. It is nearly impossible to cover a topic so dense in such a compressed manner. Nevertheless, the story can be summarized as follows. The effect of dietary fat on heart disease, cancer, and other diseases common in the West took center stage in the 1950s, and it has been treated as a high-priority research topic ever since.[31,60-65] The alleged role of dietary fat in the causation of these diseases was first interpreted in reference to the *total amount* of dietary fat consumed. The discussion then shifted to focus more on *type* of fat than *amount*, and on saturated fat specifically, which garnered attention as "bad fat." However, the assumption that saturated fats increase serum cholesterol and risk for heart disease has drawn significant criticism; as has been asserted, "conclusive evidence establishing a link between intake of saturated fatty acids and blood cholesterol level does not exist."[49] As a consequence, various types of unsaturated fat began drawing interest.[66,67] The research of the last couple decades has focused increasingly on the effects of polyunsaturated omega-3 and omega-6 fats.[49,55]

This focus on fats has completely ignored the effect of animal protein. In point of fact, our focus on fats is a *by-product of* our refusal to focus on animal protein. Distracted by discussions of whether total fat forecasts disease, or whether saturated fats are always bad, we have ignored the animal foods they are associated with and the protein those foods contain. Likewise, distracted by discussions of the goodness of unsaturated fats, and especially omega-3s, we have largely ignored their health-promoting power in *whole* plant foods and implicitly endorsed the consumption of "healthy" oils, which are not actually healthy.

Given our unwillingness to discuss animal protein, is it any wonder that the public is confused about fat? Or that we resort to simplistic good fat–bad fat arguments? Many throw up their arms in resignation and just continue eating whatever they enjoy most. To cover their bases, they buy omega-3 supplements and hope for the best. I can't help but fear for the health of these people, and for the health of our society should these trends continue.

My suggestion to combat this public confusion and distortion of facts is simple but all-encompassing. If we insist on identifying a specific cause of heart disease and other chronic metabolic diseases, rather than considering the broader dietary context, animal protein is the best culprit. Not because animal protein alone accounts for heart disease but because of the decreased consumption of heart-protective whole plant foods that accompanies its increased consumption. The consumption of animal protein is associated with many mechanisms that have adverse effects on several disease outcomes (e.g., cardiovascular disease, diabetes, cancer, and other so-called diseases of aging). It (1) increases free-radical oxidation,[68–70] (2) alters adrenal hormone activities in an unfavorable direction (increasing estrogen and testosterone),[71] (3) creates metabolic acidosis (lower body pH), (4) increases growth hormone activities (more cell division), and (5) minimizes antioxidant activities. Add to this a similar collection of mechanisms resulting from decreased consumption of plants and it becomes clear that a decision to consume animal-based protein is far more consequential than any specific recommendation pertaining to fat. But we will never confront that consumption, so long as we continue to cling to the myth of animal protein's "high quality."

OTHER SIDE EFFECTS, BEYOND NUTRITION

Our refusal to acknowledge a role for animal protein in disease formation has other consequences today, apart from contributing to the public's misunderstanding of nutrition research, and I would be remiss to ignore them here.

CONFUSION ABOUT THE CAUSE OF CANCER

The first and most obvious has already been discussed at great length in Part I: we have ignored nutrition's role in preventing and treating cancer, as well as the role of malnutrition (propelled by animal protein consumption) in promoting cancer. Instead of focusing on nutrition, cancer researchers have given their attention to environmental mutation-causing chemical carcinogens. For many years, I was somewhat influenced by this conventional wisdom. Early in my career, I had an active laboratory research program funded by NIH that investigated the role of aflatoxin (AF), a highly potent carcinogen, in the causation of primary human liver cancer. The toxin's chemical structure[72] and exceptional potency[73] were subsequently established by two groups of researchers at MIT and by my lab.[74,75] I later published a review of AF metabolism and toxicity,[76] established a laboratory in the Philippines for testing AF present in food products,[77] and developed a novel procedure for testing AF consumption in children by measuring its metabolites in the urine.[78] In 1980, I was even invited to write the lead paper on chemical carcinogens and cancer[79] in the journal of the Federation of American Societies for Experimental Biology and Medicine, the largest professional biomedical research society of its kind.

Of course, the extent to which I kept with the conventional wisdom on environmental carcinogens and cancer changed when I discovered experimental animal research, and a few correlation studies on diet and cancer in human populations, that indicated dietary protein might play a much greater role than previously imagined.[80,81] In our large 1983–1984 survey of human cancer in rural China,[82] AF exposure was recorded in three different ways, but none had a significant relationship with liver cancer mortality.[83] Instead, the chief causes of death from liver cancer were chronic infection with hepatitis B virus and consumption of animal-protein-based foods.[82] The animal protein link appeared significant even at levels of intake considered very low in the West, suggesting that animal protein intake should not merely be reduced but possibly avoided altogether.

Decades have passed since I first questioned the supposed link between human cancer and environmental chemicals like AF, and today I believe that nutrition is far more responsible for cancer than gene mutations triggered by environmental chemicals.[84] Still, for most of the science community and the lay public alike, the conventional theory emphasizing environmental chemicals remains intact. These two hypotheses—nutrition versus gene mutation—offer significantly different approaches to cancer prevention and treatment. They shape our perspectives in numerous ways. Whereas the nutrition theory suggests that the food we eat can control the formation and subsequent effects of mutations, even after they have occurred, the gene mutation theory instead encourages a perpetual search for cancer-causing agents and suggests that we are helpless to react once those mutations take over.

The gene mutation theory of cancer is, in my view, premised on an exceedingly simplistic, superficial, and damaging understanding of mutations and their causes. A mutation is what happens when a chemical or other factor (called a mutagen) permanently damages a cell's DNA, impacting gene function. When a mutated cell divides, producing daughter cells, this DNA damage is passed on to those new cells. The odds of reversing course through a back-mutation are thought to be extremely slim.

However, Nature has developed at least two mechanisms to keep this process under control. The first repairs the initial DNA damage before the cell divides. Occasionally, though, this may not occur in time, and the damaged DNA is passed on to the daughter cells. Thankfully, Nature has yet another backup: she recruits the immune system to produce "natural killer cells," which have an uncanny ability to selectively recognize and destroy these newly mutated cells before they proliferate into cancer (or some other disease).

These safeguards are, of course, not perfect. If the cell environment is fertile for cell division and growth, as in the consumption of animal protein and its many nutrient partners, millions of cells eventually accumulate despite these mechanisms and form cancer. (And although I learned this process primarily through our research on cancer, I am convinced that this same process applies, in principle, to the development of many diseases. While our bodies have mechanisms that, in the right nutritional environment, are effective in fighting those diseases, those mechanisms become hampered or overwhelmed by poor nutrition.) Unfortunately, rather than focusing on enhancing the body's natural mechanisms for dealing with mutations, or changing people's behaviors that proliferate cell division, the cancer research community focuses virtually all of its attention and resources on the mutagens that initiate cancer.

The cancer research community, underwritten by hundreds of billions of dollars and the belief that cell mutations do not self-correct, also makes another key mistake: it bases its work on the premise that keeping these chemicals under control will prevent cancer. Reality is more complicated, and focusing exclusively on mutagenic chemicals leaves us at a serious disadvantage. These chemicals—pesticides, herbicides, industrial chemicals, food additives, and the like—are very diverse in their chemical and biological properties,[85,86] and thus may cause a wide variety of unpredictable toxicities and diseases. Not *all* chemicals that cause mutations cause cancer; neither is cancer "caused" *only* by mutagens. Various nonmutagenic food products, chemical mixtures, and procedures have also been classified as carcinogens.[87,88] Moreover, thousands of mutations, even hundreds of thousands, arise in the normal course of cell division in *each individual cell*! Determining which of them actually causes cancer is no small task, and of course excludes the fact that other factors participate in the expression of those mutations, as we saw above. Despite all of these complicating factors, the belief that the terms *mutagen* and *carcinogen* are almost interchangeable has become widespread, leading to confusion and misplaced research policy priorities.

Our fixation on the idea that cancer is mainly dependent on mutations that, once occurring, inexorably move forward compels an exclusive focus on experimentally testing environmental chemicals for their cancer-producing potential. And there are thought to be a vast number of chemicals to test. During the past sixty to seventy years, various testing methods have been developed to assess an estimated 80,000* suspect chemicals. Since the early '70s, however, the primary carcinogen-testing program has been the experimental animal bioassay program, which determines cancer potential by testing suspect chemicals on living systems, most often on rats and mice, but also on isolated cultures of specific cells grown under laboratory conditions.[79,89,90] Developed jointly by two institutes of the National Institutes of Health

---

* This figure of 80,000 chemicals has been widely quoted for at least forty years. Surely there are far more.

(NIH), the National Cancer Institute (NCI) and the National Institute of Environmental Health Sciences (NIEHS), this program is now operated by the interagency National Toxicology Program within the Department of Health and Human Services.[91] The animal bioassay is the core component of this toxicology program,[92,93] which has recently issued its fourteenth report on carcinogens.[94]

Unsurprisingly, with so many decades and resources already devoted to research efforts driven by the gene mutation theory, no one wants to hear a nutrition-centered perspective, especially one that questions animal protein. To declare animal protein as a cause of cancer, and a more influential one than environmental chemicals, is to undermine the premise and previous efforts of an entire field. Furthermore, it would undermine many future research efforts, a sensitive subject given how many jobs are currently on the line.

Back in the '80s, I was invited by professional organizations to share my views on the animal bioassay programs, twice in the US (by the NIEHS in Research Triangle Park, North Carolina, and at its laboratory in Jefferson, Arkansas) and once in Lyon, France (by the International Agency of Research on Cancer of the United Nations' World Health Organization). In each case, although my interpretation of the science was never challenged, I experienced a serious and stubborn reluctance to even entertain a role for nutrition in cancer. In North Carolina, the program director bluntly told me in front of a large audience that changes in the program mission would not happen unless I could "convince the White House."

The sad reality is that our approach to cancer, fundamentally, does not rely on basic science. Too many research pathologists' careers depend on the assumption that single, identifiable chemicals are the main causes of cancer. This is the case in both public and private laboratories. In addition, cancer has been framed since its discovery as an aggressive and nonreversible disease, meaning that once it is diagnosed, and especially after it spreads from its origin to distant tissues, it cannot be reversed, only destroyed. The supposed lethality of the disease is terrifying, to say the least, and the intensity of our search for identifiable cancer-causing chemicals is driven by that terror. I believe both of these reasons help to explain why the animal bioassay program has enjoyed high-priority status for so long.

To make matters even trickier, though, the bioassay program is already clouded in some ethical controversy due to its reliance on experimental animal testing.[95–97] Public authorities have justified the program's use of animals in the name of a laudable goal—searching for solutions to human cancer—but these authorities aren't interested in inviting further controversy by backpedaling or implicating some of our favorite foods in cancer causation, regardless of chemical contamination. A perfect illustration of this monstrous dilemma concerns casein, the aforementioned animal-based protein of cow's milk. In animal studies, casein causes a remarkably potent cancer response, even at common levels of consumption. Were it to be tested under the specifications of that animal bioassay program, it would undoubtedly be the most powerful chemical carcinogen ever discovered! So, too, would other animal proteins. I can hardly think of a better illustration of how our celebrated "science" is failing us.

The animal bioassay program is only one example—albeit a large and significant one—of conventional cancer research efforts stemming from the gene mutation theory. The work of genetic scientists, too, would be threatened by a greater focus on nutrition. The Human Genome Project, for example, has had an enormous impact on cancer research by discovering many details of cancer formation on the genetic level—identifying, for example, which genes or gene products are associated with which type of cancer—and many have heralded it as the greatest research project ever undertaken.[98] All of these efforts have further reinforced the sacrosanct belief that cancer is a "genetic disease," as NCI spotlights on its website.[99]

Now, I don't mean to suggest that environmental chemicals and genes play *no* role in cancer formation. It would be incorrect to deny the link. But the story, as we've seen, is not nearly as straightforward as most seem to think.

Last, consider the following, which further undermines the theory that cancer is a genetic disease caused by environmental chemicals:

1. The aforementioned animal bioassay program is only impressive if one assumes that the same chemicals toxic to experimental animals are also toxic to humans. Unless human population studies can show associations consistent with those in experimental animals,

such species-to-species extrapolation is as much a leap of faith as it is an example of sound science. As of now, population studies, when compared with the evidence on nutrition, show almost no evidence of causal associations of environmental chemicals with human cancers.

2. In laboratory studies, modest changes in nutrient intake can cause substantial changes in cancer outcomes initiated by known carcinogens.[39] In our laboratory, we repeatedly showed the ability of diet to modify the development of liver cancer initiated by AF, both by promoting its growth with a high-animal-protein diet and repressing its growth with a low-animal-protein diet. (Incidentally, given that I have just critiqued the animal bioassay program for extrapolating results from nonhuman species, I should point out that human population studies do show associations when it comes to nutrition and cancer consistent with my lab's findings. I will discuss this research in greater depth in Part III.)

3. Although mutagenic chemicals may be experimentally associated with certain cancers, when administered at a very high dose (as in the case of AF and liver cancer) along with a cancer-promotive diet, none show a breadth of effect as impressive as the association between nutrition and cancer. Poor nutrition is not associated with only one type of cancer, but with the vast majority.

4. It is doubtful whether additional mutations triggered by environmental chemicals cause a cancer response when our mutation burden is already so significant. Remember, thousands of mutations can and do exist in every cell. Without a nutritional stimulus, it's unclear whether extra mutations produce a response. In our experimental animal research, we found that increasing the carcinogen dose caused a linear increase in the formation of mutations, as expected, but that those mutations only developed into cancer when promoted by animal protein.[100–102] In the absence of appropriate nutritional stimulus, increasing mutations do not appear to develop into cancers.[103]

Given all of this, I reject the common understanding of cancer as primarily determined by toxin-initiated genetic mutations. The pathway from environmental chemicals to genes to genetic mutations to cancer-cell growth to diagnosable cancer is appealing in its simplicity, but insufficient and far too narrowly focused. Moreover, it blatantly ignores the possibility of individuals themselves being able to control cancer. By ignoring nutrition's role in the promotion of cancer, a role that has been demonstrated in both observational human studies and experimental animal studies, we ignore our best chance at preventing the disease and disregard all personal agency. This negligence is obviously abhorrent when it comes to human health, but it does rather conveniently allow us to continue enjoying foods containing that dear "high quality" driver nutrient, animal protein.

ENVIRONMENTAL CONCERNS

In addition to its effects on human health, our refusal to address the harm of animal protein in a substantive way has had a profound effect on planetary health. I speak now of environmental chemicals and big agribusiness not as a cause of cancer, but as a threat to our planet and the life it supports. Indicators suggest that we are in the midst of an environmental crisis, quickly developing into an environmental calamity. According to the latest climate reports, "to keep warming under 1.5°C, countries will have to cut global CO_2 emissions 45 percent below 2010 levels by 2030" and reach carbon neutrality (balancing emissions with CO_2 intake by plants) by 2050.[104] To reach this goal, we must overcome our addiction to fossil fuels and take a serious look at how our economic and academic systems obfuscate the truth. No amount of profit could ever justify this universal self-harm.

With regard to species loss, we are in the midst of a mass extinction caused by human action. According to mathematical models published in *Nature*, species extinction rates can increase exponentially as a result of co-extinction: "climate change and human activity are dooming species at an unprecedented rate via a plethora of direct and indirect, often synergic mechanisms. Among these, primary extinction driven by environmental change could be just the tip of the iceberg."[105] Some estimates suggest that Earth is losing animal species anywhere from 1,000 to 10,000 times the natural rate.[106] Nowhere are these trends more alarming than in insect populations:[107] 41 percent of all insect species have seen steep declines over the past decade, and scientists now estimate that 40 percent of the roughly 30 million insect species on Earth are under threat of extinction. The order of insects known as Lepidoptera, which includes butterflies, has declined by 53 percent, while those in the order Orthoptera, which include grasshoppers and crickets, have declined by approximately 50 percent. Although many people of my generation may speak of changes they've witnessed in their lifetimes, the frightening truth is that these developments are only accelerating. To hear even my grandchildren talk about changes they have noticed within their short lifetimes—to think that they may someday not come into contact with grasshoppers in their natural setting—is astonishing.

Environmental impact assessments are relatively new phenomena that have aided us in understanding to what extent various activities are affecting the environment. The first of these assessments of livestock that gained traction publicly was a 2006 report from the UN's Food and Agriculture Organization in which they declared livestock responsible for 18 percent of greenhouse gas emissions, more than all of human transport put together. This was later recalculated by the Worldwatch Institute in 2009 to be 51 percent,[108] following a 1996 alert published by Lester Brown,[109] and an even earlier suggestion by Hindhede[110]—more than all other human-made factors combined. Although these numbers are still subject to contentious debate, we can no longer deny that the rearing and raising of livestock has contributed to climate change significantly and disproportionately. If we want to address emissions, it is absolutely critical that we address livestock production.

In short, the uncomfortable fact that so many seem intent on ignoring is that these trends are connected to the food we eat and the way we produce it. Enjoying foods further up the food chain, especially animal foods, requires more farmland and resources. This results in the destruction of forests around the world; the trampling of fields beneath the wheels of massive tractors and harvesting machines; the treatment and tilling of land with an eye always on short-term profit rather than ecological longevity and health; and the use of hormones to speed the production of meat, milk, and eggs from animals whose lives have shrunk to fit within the confines of a hell that's half prison, half factory.* We howl about environmental chemicals in the cancer research community, but dump vast numbers of these chemicals into the food system. On a superficial level, we do this to fight off weeds and pests, in the name of higher immediate yields. But at what cost? How much longer can we wage war against the environment, and for what gain? How much longer do we wish to survive?

Malnutrition, characterized by a diet *high in animal protein* and processed foods, and therefore also low in nutritious plant foods, seems to me a far greater threat to human health than the environmental chemicals discussed in the previous section. But that doesn't mean environmental chemicals are a nonissue. To raise alarm about those chemicals in one arena, while simultaneously worsening our environment's chemical burden in another, just to produce more of the high-protein foods contributing to disease . . . are we really so committed to testing the limits of our delusions?

Our widespread use of the weed killer Roundup is perhaps the best example of this contradiction. In 1987 it was the seventeenth most used pesticide, but by 2011 it reached number one worldwide.[111] Its active ingredient is the herbicide glyphosate, and in commercial operations it is mostly used on crops genetically modified to resist it. This allows farmers to spray Roundup indiscriminately, selectively killing weeds without destroying the modified crop. In the days before Roundup, my brothers and I all earned money for college by driving self-propelled, grain-harvesting combines during the summertime (yes, we participated in the agricultural revolution, too). In some cases, we could not avoid "harvesting" some weed seeds along with the grain, but this was not considered an issue unless the harvested grain was to be used as seed for a new crop. Nearly fifty years later I began to see more fields of grain without weeds and learned how it was accomplished. The miracle combination of herbicide and genetic modification had arrived.

It is the height of arrogance to believe we can control and bend nature to our iron will, but we are always testing those heights. We assert that we can eradicate pests and weeds with chemicals, but we are not only eradicating pests and weeds. In point of fact, we are waging chemical warfare against the natural world. While the plants may be genetically modified to withstand

---

* Milking cows once lived an average of fifteen to twenty years; now it's closer to five.

the effects of glyphosate, the insects and other animals who unavoidably come in contact with the chemical do not. Sadly, pollinators have no sway in Congress. There is no coalition of bees fighting in Washington, DC, for their and our survival. Meanwhile, evidence has emerged to suggest that glyphosate has a variety of toxicities for humans, too. As of May 2019, its maker, Bayer, faced lawsuits from more than 13,000 plaintiffs for Roundup-related poisoning in the United States.[107]

Ultimately, no matter which subject we turn to in this book, humanity's tendency toward myopia never fails to rear its ugly head. Our reliance on targeted chemicals in agriculture is disturbingly similar to the chemotherapist of old's reliance on colloidal lead therapy, as described in Part I; in both cases we have relied on simplistic strategies (almost always unproven and with unknown consequences!) for dealing with complex challenges and systems. It's as if we have committed ourselves to missing the greater context of things, time and time again.

Perhaps this is just our way of coping with cognitive dissonance, the psychological phenomenon arising from inconsistent thoughts, beliefs, and attitudes. One minute we purport to care about health, development, and safety; in the next we celebrate activities that damage health, development, and safety. We purport to care about individual freedom to access health care and information, especially in the United States, but only until health care and information threaten powerful interests. It seems to me that our most common response to such cognitive dissonance is to ignore the uncomfortable facts altogether, each of us burrowing deeper into the caverns of our own denial. Just as we cope with dissonance when it comes to the destruction of our bodies and our "health care" system, so too is it with the destruction of the environment: a carefully aligned blindfold, befitting a wildly misaligned people.

I've spoken to many environmental protection groups, including the public support groups of the US Environmental Protection Agency (EPA), EarthSave, and the Sierra Club. Unfortunately, according to the people who invite me, these organizations are not interested in hearing about a role for nutrition in human health when dealing with environmental catastrophe. On one occasion, while attending a small discussion group of environmental enthusiasts, I heard the director of the Natural Resources Defense Council

(NRDC) say that it would be difficult, if not suicidal, for his organization to advocate to their donors that diet might be important in resolving the climate crisis. He explained that NRDC donors would strongly object, even though convincing evidence now shows that livestock farming is a major cause of climate change.[108,112] In other words, the NRDC was making a judgment on behalf of its three million members, rather than giving them the information and letting them decide what to do with it. At best, such a policy is paternalistic and patronizing. At worst, it ensures that the organization will continue marching toward the same fate its director wanted to avoid—death by suicide—for if we don't address this existential threat fully and responsibly, our fates are sealed.

I wouldn't suggest that the NRDC is an unusual case, or that the people working there have poor intentions. This is not a case of blatant corruption. They have actively supported legislation to help reduce the amount of environmental chemicals pumped into our environment, an effort I view as valuable in and of itself. They also encourage the public to pitch in: bike whenever possible to reduce emissions, take shorter showers, recycle, and so forth. But when it comes to nutrition and the systemic issues related to how food is produced, they keep their distance. I suspect this is the case for the same reasons many cancer research institutions avoid discussing nutrition: the scope of their advocacy is limited by the confines of a prohibitive system. In both cases, our negligence in failing to factor in the effect of animal protein has done profound damage.

To end this section on a high note, I'd emphasize that agriculture presents a tremendous opportunity to undo many of the problems facing the environment today. Consider the opportunity cost of producing livestock. Opportunity cost is defined as the loss of potential gain from other alternatives when one alternative is chosen. For livestock, the opportunity cost is whatever might be gained by *not* raising livestock. Based on all the evidence I've cited and the dire state of things as they are, I believe it would be no exaggeration to say that the opportunity cost of raising livestock may be the continuance of life on this planet as we know it.

Consider that right now on our planet, approximately 70 billion animals are raised as livestock for human consumption every year.[113] Stop for a moment and consider the immense resources necessary to house, feed, slaughter, and transport all of these animals. This system is inherently inefficient. When one considers potential alternatives, we can see the enormous realms of possibility. Consider also that 45 percent of all tillable land is currently used for livestock and feed. Despite that, only 20 percent of all calories consumed by humans come from animal-based foods. That means 80 percent of all calories consumed by humans come from plant-based foods. And how much of the tillable land is being used to provide those calories? *Only 5 percent.*[114]

Here we have a case of blatant inefficiency. Imagine if we took the land currently used for livestock and feed, which is now contributing to climate change, and instead reforested it and revitalized the degraded soil. In doing so, we would limit all the pollution related to livestock production, including the groundwater pollution created by the two billion tons of feces produced by livestock every year and the fossil fuel–based fertilizers used to grow feed for livestock, both of which are creating dead zones globally.[115] We would also create one of the world's largest carbon sinks.

The potential benefits of such changes are truly monumental, and here's the clincher—we would be healthier as a result. What is good for the planet is good for us.

IN DEFENSE OF *USEFUL* CONTROVERSY

Each of the topics discussed here has become fixed in the public mindset. Each has been the subject of confusion and misinformation. Dysfunction is the default today when it comes to nutrition, and these debates have kept us stranded in the superficial. To avoid a deeper understanding of nutrition that threatens industry (but would also save lives), we have mistakenly attached ourselves to other dietary factors, in effect looking for scapegoats for our nutrition ignorance.

We made fat the villain, resulting in a massive market for low-fat dairy and lean cuts of meats, and advertised these low-fat alternatives as a healthy way to enjoy our favorite foods. We blamed saturated fat and dietary cholesterol for the rise in heart disease, despite evidence linking animal protein to the disease, and fought this fabricated problem by setting limits on cholesterol intake and developing cholesterol-lowering drugs and procedures that fail to deal with the underlying problem. We laid the blame for cancer entirely on environmental chemicals and their ability to mutate genes, ignoring the empowering prospect of controlling the expression of mutations through healthful eating. And then, despite laying the blame on environmental chemicals, we kept dumping chemicals into the environment anyway, and increased greenhouse gas emissions, just so that we could continue to enjoy our favorite foods. All the while, we encouraged the consumption of "high-quality" animal protein, an oxymoron and relic originating a century ago, and set irresponsible and immoral "upper safe limits" for its consumption.

Putting animal protein off limits and dismissing any evidence that disagrees with the status quo is a great way to encourage confusion, but it's also effective for avoiding *useful* controversy and preventing change. The superficial, noisy hubbub surrounding cholesterol and fats is as much a sign of this avoidance as is the absence of nutrition from conversations about cancer and the environment.

In this light, the dismissal of the WFPB diet and its supporting evidence is a way to avoid changing our beliefs about animal protein. In this case, avoiding controversy, avoiding change, is not a good thing. The present system requires disruption. So long as we remain wedded to animal protein and obsessed with related myths, debates, and diversions, we will not achieve an understanding of nutrition's full potential, but neither will we even know what nutrition's full potential can be. The prevailing narrative is one we must move past.

However, even if we were to wake up tomorrow accepting nutrition's essential relationship to health, most people would still be confused about what good nutrition is, as evidenced by the examples provided in the last two chapters. Said another way, they don't know what they don't know.

There is, in my view, more than sufficient evidence for us to say what good nutrition is. I have already introduced some of this evidence and will be elaborating further in the next section of this book. But the problem we face—the third piece of controversy in this puzzle—is that the evidence in support of a WFPB diet challenges conventional attitudes about *evidence* itself, just as it challenges conventional attitudes about *disease care* and *nutrition*. In a critical sense, this evidence challenges the entire scientific enterprise and the way it studies and deliberates on biological phenomena. It challenges the "science" by which we examine ourselves—the "science" by which we describe ourselves as mechanical assemblages of molecules. It challenges, in other words, our very means of explaining life, our failure to capture and experience the beauty of Nature.

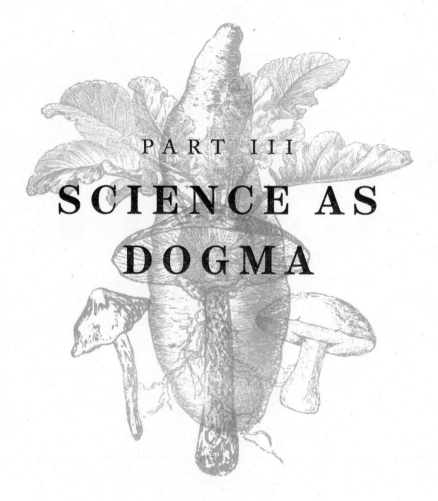

PART III

SCIENCE AS DOGMA

CHAPTER SEVEN

A RADICAL
CHALLENGE TO
SCIENCE

*It seems sometimes that people . . . fill their eyes with things
seen microscopically in order to not see macroscopically.*
—Marilyn Frye

The word *radical* comes from the Latin *radix*, meaning root. Consider some of the common contexts in which *radical* is used: radical social reform seeks to address the fundamentals of our society; the concept of radical acceptance, touted by various life philosophies, encourages us to embrace things as they are, not only superficially but also at their roots; and any radical revolution that does not address the root causes of our systems is, well, perhaps not as radical as advertised. Likewise, a radical critique is one concerned with the fundamentals of its subject, and a radical challenge is one that confronts its subject's fundamentals.

We have at this point explored two important ways in which the whole food, plant-based (WFPB) diet radically challenges the status quo. The first radical challenge is aimed at our beliefs about disease and health, and our power over them. For instance, it challenges our belief that diseases are meant to be discrete—in their naming, their pathology, and their management. Accordingly, we believe that given sufficient information, diseases can be technically and specifically managed. This motivates us to discover ever more discrete details on pathology and management—the purview of modern science—and encourages ever more specific, isolated solutions, both in identification of causes and refinement of treatments. This may seem fair and reasonable enough, but there is a cost. It tends to lead us astray from the concept of interconnectedness, the essence of nature. The WFPB diet, the effectiveness of which is explained by the interconnectedness of nature, is therefore ignored. The evidence supporting the WFPB diet challenges these and many other historically entrenched, institutionally enforced attitudes about disease and its causes, and in so doing challenges both our understanding and approach to a wide spectrum of conventional disease treatment.

The second radical challenge that the WFPB diet poses is to the field of nutrition, which has tended toward confusion and misapplication since at least the mid-nineteenth century. The WFPB diet clarifies nutrition, collates dietary advice for the vast majority of people into two very simple instructions (consume whole foods and avoid animal foods), and empowers the individual. In its push for clarity, simplicity, and accessibility, it challenges nutrition's long-standing, dominant patterns. Moreover, it challenges long-held nutrition science myths, especially our veneration of animal protein. By extension, it challenges ongoing debates about fat, cholesterol, and more—or rather, it simplifies these debates out of existence.

We have now arrived at a third reason that the WFPB diet is controversial, and this is perhaps the most radical of them all: the WFPB diet and its supporting evidence radically challenge our attitudes toward *science* and *evidence* themselves. This challenge is inherent in the evidence I am speaking of in support of a WFPB diet because that evidence doesn't fit within conventional parameters. By this, I do not in any way mean that the WFPB diet is supported by "bad" evidence; on the contrary, it is supported by a very impressive body of scientifically sound evidence. Rather, it does not fit within the bounds of what many scientists designate as the "best" science and the "best" evidence. The problem is that these designations are based on human value judgments. The science community has long favored *certain* kinds of evidence, *certain* methodologies, and *certain* narrow interpretations, and the evidence in favor of a WFPB diet does not always cohere with these. In short, the WFPB diet forces us to rethink our notions of what is "good" evidence.

THE SUBJECTIVITY OF "OBJECTIVE" SCIENCE

In no way should my critique of these value judgments be taken as an argument against all of traditional science. I am not suggesting we should chuck out the scientific method, or distrust its aims. Modern science has without a doubt added tremendous value to our lives, and the "objective" scientist's ideal of hermetically sealed truths is not without merit. What I am suggesting, rather, is a more nuanced application of these methods.

The "real world" isn't as easily controlled as a double-blind experiment conducted in a laboratory setting, and neither are the activities surrounding the present conduct of science: competition for research funding, the politics of academia, policy development, and any of the other arenas in which scientists might have occasion to spar. The "real world" is rife with human error. Trying to make sense of this human error is not an easy task, but we should at least admit that it exists. And the way in which we selectively celebrate certain kinds of evidence and certain research methodologies, while ignoring or devaluing others, is just one example of how science can become susceptible to human error.

I am not suggesting that this is an outright conspiracy perpetrated by the world's scientists, but that it is a blind spot and a shortcoming. To give just one example (I'll have more later), our outsized celebration of the double-blind, placebo-controlled study, often called the "gold standard" in intervention-based studies, is not always warranted, and especially not in the field of nutrition.

It is an excellent study design for testing pills, because that involves changing only one variable at a time, but not for testing an entire dietary lifestyle, which contains countless variables whose ever-changing relationships and outcomes are impossible to fully control for. Accordingly, our selective appreciation for this kind of study speaks to a selective appreciation for pharmaceutical solutions and a selective dismissal of nuanced nutritional solutions.

I am not suggesting that double-blind, placebo-controlled studies are "bad" in any way—just that they are not always best, and that our celebration of this study design is mandated not by any superhuman authority, but by our own fallible judgment. The appeal of this study design is obvious and understandable. That we should be drawn to the simplest, tidiest study designs is not surprising. It seems to remove, as much as possible, the biased influence of the human observer. It also reflects a centuries-long drift toward reductionist science, arising from the mid-nineteenth-century's local theory of disease causation.

What I hope to do in this third part of the book is challenge those who would critique, dismiss, or ignore the WFPB diet and its supporting evidence on the grounds that it has not been proven by the most rigorous standards of science today. I hope to clarify that these standards are not set in stone. We need to ask, especially when it comes to nutrition, *what is good science, what is good evidence,* and *who determines these standards?*

The answer to the final question, as we have seen in each of the two previous sections, is often institutions, which are subject to the same biases as their founders and their society. Recall some of the ways in which the science of health has been subjected to the biases of its gatekeepers:

- Of the eleven charter members of the American Association for Cancer Research (AACR), none had any background whatsoever in nutrition. The subsequent research funded by that organization, both then and now, has tended toward the preferred treatments of its founders, especially surgery.
- At the seminal 1926 American Cancer Society (ACS) conference at Lake Mohonk, the roster of speakers excluded pioneers of epidemiology (Frederick Hoffman) and critics of radiotherapy (Charles Gibson).

- At the same conference, Professor of Clinical Surgery Howard Lilienthal blatantly misrepresented Gibson's research in order to celebrate his own favored cancer treatment: surgery.
- In a 1926 study published by Copeman and Greenwood, sponsored by the British Empire Cancer Campaign (BECC), the authors rediagnosed death certificates and discarded data when it disagreed with their expected findings.
- The research of Russell Chittenden and Irvine Fisher, both Yale professors who studied diet and athletic performance, was quickly forgotten, as was the publication of nine manuscripts in 1983 investigating the role of animal protein in the progression of atherosclerosis.[1]

Of course, these are very blatant examples, and perhaps some of them are dated, but that does not mean that similar biases and consequences do not persist. And though today's examples may not always reek as obviously of foul play, they may be even more dangerous, for they are entrenched deeper than ever in our institutions, celebrated again and again as "the best of science," and we seem to have forgotten that alternatives exist.

REDUCTIONIST SCIENCE AND STANDARDS OF EVIDENCE

Despite an increasing amount of research conducted during the last century, not only in nutrition but also in other specialties of health and medicine, it is difficult to say whether our collective wisdom in this sphere of science has progressed. Scientists often squabble over extremely minute details of their respective, siloed fields. Indeed, it is the minute details that almost exclusively consume us, a phenomenon called *scientific reductionism*. This focus on reductionism is easy to ignore because it is everywhere, but also hard to miss, once you're looking for it. And reductionism's sole focus on details has many consequences.

The vast majority of research findings during the past few decades belong to this camp of scientific reductionism. This includes science that investigates minute details in isolation; science that believes the world can be understood by mapping all its component parts; science directed at the accumulation of information over the synthesis of that information into practicable wisdom; and science that is compartmentalized and often poorly communicated, both with other scientific disciplines and with the public.

Reductionism is the "good" science of today. It is the unrivaled, dominant mode of understanding the world. And the central figure of this reductionist system is the specialist: the protagonist of modern science, the seeker of splintered truth. And indeed, when reductionism is the dominant mode of understanding the world, it follows that specialists would play the most substantial part in scientific discovery. By always drilling toward greater precision and detail, our society is always requiring further specialization; the specialist is the inevitable by-product. This is not, on its face, a tragedy. But missing from this scheme is any counterbalance. We have isolated expertise, but in the process sacrificed context. As a result, the usefulness of our expertise is limited, separate not only from the ivory towers of other specialists, but also from the rest of society.

And what do reductionist specialists today consider to be "good" evidence on topics of diet and health? Published in 1965,[2] Sir Bradford Hill's famous list of nine criteria for evaluating the quality of evidence provides an excellent starting point. These are the criteria that nutrition and human health researchers most often use to determine the value of new evidence, whether consciously or subconsciously; the more clearly evidence fulfills these criteria, and the more criteria it fulfills, the stronger it is considered to be.

Criteria for Reliability of Evidence

Criterion	Explanation
1. Strength	When there exist strong associations (e.g., a ten-fold size of effect versus a two-fold size of effect) . . . they are generally viewed as more reliable.
2. Consistency	When the findings of a hypothesis by different authors and different study designs agree . . .

3.	Specificity	When size of effect and significance of a single causal factor is much greater than for other factors ...
4.	Temporality	When the cause precedes the effect ...
5.	Gradient	When the effect increases with the exposure, or "dose" ...
6.	Plausibility	When a hypothetical cause can be explained mechanistically ...
7.	Coherence	When the findings of a study align with other generally known facts ...
8.	Experiment	When carefully designed experimental tests of a hypothesis agree ...
9.	Analogy	When analogies or similarities exist between the observed cause-and-effect relationship and other well-accepted associations ...

And what kinds of research studies are conducted? It should come as no surprise that the most respected are those with the most razor-sharp focus, which allow the researchers as much control over the research conditions as is possible. Five main types of research studies are used in nutrition research:

- *Intervention studies,* which include the double-blind randomized controlled trial mentioned previously (in which neither researchers nor randomly assigned subjects know whether they are in the control or treatment groups), are those in which subjects receive some kind of intervention, such as a pill.
- *Cohort studies* are those in which dietary and health information is collected on a large group of individuals for a period of time before disease occurrence; then statistical analysis of the effects of possible disease-causing factors is undertaken. (These studies are considered *prospective* if the dietary information is recorded before the event occurs or *retrospective* if the dietary information is recalled after the fact.)
- *Observational studies* compare the disease rates and dietary practices of groups of people (villages, nations, etc.), which may or may not yield *correlations.* Observational studies are often described as "snapshots in time."

- *Laboratory studies* search for biochemical and physiological explanations for how certain dietary factors may promote or inhibit disease, often with experimental animals.
- Last, *case-control* studies compare people with disease (cases) to otherwise similar people without disease (controls), to assess what differences might explain the presence of disease in one group but not the other.

Unsurprisingly, under present conditions, the most highly valued of these evidence criteria and research studies, intervention studies, are also the most useful for reductionist research questions, such as in the study of drugs.

I don't list these study types now to bore you, but rather to set the stage more fully. What we have here is a collection of useful tools for assessing the world we live in. But there has come to be an imbalance in how we use these tools. Always, we are applying them in a way that reinforces the broad consensus that scientific reductionism is the best and only appropriate path forward.

REDUCTIONISM IN ACTION

Of course, reductionist techniques are frequently welcome and useful. One would be hard-pressed to name any major breakthroughs of the past century in anatomy, chemistry, physics, or biology that did not benefit in some way from reductionist tools or philosophies. Working with minute details is often critically important. I certainly hope that our aeronautical engineers, who design the machines that I so often trust to carry me at altitudes thousands of feet in the sky, are trained to do just that.

The problem, then, is not with reductionism itself, but rather the circumstances that arise when reductionism is the only game in town. While it may be well attuned to the study of minute component parts within Nature, the ever-narrowing focus of reductionism is incompatible with any halfway-useful understanding of Nature as a whole. Said another way: as useful as reductionism may be for describing parts of the world, it is not sufficient for understanding the world. It is a zoom lens capable of producing miraculous, even beautiful, discoveries, but without employing other perspectives, we are limiting ourselves.

Central to the concept of reductionism is the assumption that the world is made up of parts, each with their own distinct edges, and that by studying those parts in isolation, we can glean some truth about the whole from which they come. But the fact of Nature is that nothing exists in isolation. Every single "part" of the world that reductionist science could possibly analyze, from aortas to enzymes to protons, exists within a larger context. Were they not part of that larger contextual system, then they would not be worth describing as parts, for they would be rendered meaningless (it is these parts' context that gives them meaning!). Moreover, each of these distinct "things" contains within it a seemingly infinite number of integrative systems, nested like Russian dolls. To rely on reductionism alone, rather than using it in alignment with other approaches, is to approach these parts and consider them in great detail, but without any understanding of the interconnectivity of our infinite, intertwined worlds.

You might be wondering about the practical implications of this imbalance, thinking that some of this discussion sounds rather academic or philosophical. Perhaps someday long ago I would have made a similar point. But now, after decades in nutrition science, I have seen the real-world consequences of reductionist dominance over the research enterprise.

My perspective on this point admittedly relies on my own experience and the experience of colleagues, but it's no small amount of experience. I've participated in the research enterprise for decades, from top to bottom. I've been on both sides of the research application table, receiving decades' worth of public funding and reviewing more research applications submitted by other scientists than I can count. Plus, I never would have been able to receive such funding, or even get my career off the ground, if I had not shown a willingness and ability to work within the reductionist paradigm. I've also been a member of expert panels that use research findings to advise on public policy. From these experiences, I know that certain research proposals are dismissed out of hand because they do not focus enough on highly specific details of nutrient function. Applications for nonreductionist research—that is, research that acknowledges and considers the real-world complexity of whole foods, with their nutrients consumed intact and in combination, rather than single nutrients in controlled settings—is derided for having a lack of focus. When I sat on review panels, I remember such applications being called "fishing expeditions" or "shotgun approaches."

The study design a researcher chooses depends on a few different factors: whether it is intended as a human population study, whether a laboratory is needed, whether requirements for human study can be approved, available funding, and so forth. Other factors influencing a researcher's chosen study design include whether they are a clinician who works with patients, whether they have an adequately equipped research laboratory, and whether they have or can get access to data on large populations. However, the finer details of a researcher's study, regardless of that study's broader design, are shaped, almost subconsciously, by our innate tendency to search for specific causes and specific mechanisms for specific diseases. Often this is useful, but this assumption also steers us away from thinking about the thirty-thousand-foot perspective.

This exclusive dominance of reductionism, not just in research funding but in the interpretation of findings, also has numerous consequences on the way in which science is communicated to the public. Among professionals and the public alike, many are tethered to an overly simplistic understanding of the scientific research enterprise, which includes an overly simplistic understanding of how to communicate what has been learned. We seem to think that good research involves doing an experiment and letting the results "speak for themselves," rather than interpreting them within a larger context. The idea of letting results speak for themselves is great in theory, but because many research studies contradict one another, interpreting the greater context of things is absolutely essential. This may sound elementary, and it really should be, but too many of us have lost sight of the need for interpretation and the existence of that greater context. We have focused more upon discovering more and more details, and not on making sense of them.

Experiments are considered best when they provide black-and-white answers that either confirm or deny our beliefs. In the search for such stark objectivity, we are drawn to the simplest research designs: randomized controlled trials in which a testable agent either has or does not have an effect. The results are then accepted as *facts*, rather than *suggestions for future research* (which is how all research findings should be regarded). Resulting from this system is a sea of highly specific, technical details and particular observations, removed from the context of our observable world. The consequent disconnect between public knowledge and scientific research is unsurprising, as is the confusion and controversy that the public has to contend with—especially when it comes to understanding what to eat. Examples from chapter six illustrate this confusion and controversy well, especially the debates surrounding fat and cholesterol. It is very easy to find contradicting research results when the most celebrated research focuses on isolated nutrients out of context.

And so, reductionism in action has a tremendous impact on the scientific enterprise at every level. From its funding to its design to its production to its publication to its communication, nearly all research today is influenced by the values of reductionism. But perhaps you will recall that I earlier introduced the term *scientific reductionism* as a "camp." I did so deliberately, to suggest that there is another possible approach to science as we have come to know it—an alternate perspective. This perspective I call *wholism*, a concept derived, at its simplest, from that millennium-old adage "The whole is greater than the sum of its parts."

WHOLISM

Let me begin by briefly defining wholism (the primary topic of my second book, *Whole*) in reference to nutrition. First, there are a virtually infinite number and variety of substances in food that help promote health and disease. The few dozen named nutrients with which we are familiar are nowhere near a comprehensive list. There could easily be hundreds of thousands of phytochemicals in plants with nutrient-like properties. Second, these substances act in a highly dynamic way. They interact endlessly with each other, within tens of trillions of cells, and change within nanoseconds. Third, the body's metabolism—the complete assembly of all of these dynamic interactions—is as controlled as a symphony. It perpetually strives for a thrifty life and the prevention of disease by conserving and distributing energy, defending against foreign agents, and removing and regenerating cells. And, the overarching fourth—there is a power managing this symphony that goes by the name "Nature."

A brief overview of the difference between reductionism and wholism, and the relationship between them, is also crucial if we are to appreciate the full extent of the controversy generated by the WFPB diet and its supporting evidence. First, I'd like to point out that there need not be any tension or conflict between wholism and reductionism. The two are not mutually exclusive; rather, wholism encompasses reductionism. I should also say that I deliberately spell the counterbalancing *wholism* with a "w" to distinguish it from *holism*, which tows behind it a heavy religious connotation and turns off many scientists as a result. When many people read the phrase *holistic science*, they immediately translate it inside their heads to *pseudoscience*. Holism reminds them of New Age belief systems not to be taken seriously. The science that I am describing, on the other hand, is distinct from any religious connotations and should be judged on its own merits, not by any dogma—neither that of religion, nor that of the reductionist scientists who believe there is only one way to study and understand the world.

Given that it encompasses but does not refute reductionism, wholism in the sciences does not prohibit the continued funding or publication of reductionist research. I hardly think I'm speaking dangerously when I say that we may benefit from both, but this is definitely a minority opinion. As a member of a research-grant review panel for the NIH's National Cancer Institute (NCI) in the 1970s and '80s, I reviewed many applications for funding in which applicants proposed a more wholistic approach to cancer research (e.g., proposing to study the effects of a wider array of causal factors). Some of these would indeed have benefited from a clearer focus or purpose, but others were very focused and in fact more aligned with a true understanding of chemistry and biology (which is far more complex than many reductionist research proposals account for). That proposals such as these are invariably dismissed is a troubling indication of how deeply entrenched reductionism has become. The introduction of wholism into our understanding of science would unsettle, even if only slightly, the long-settled belief that reductionist research is the *only* type deserving of funding. It would challenge the popular reductionist notion that large-scale correlation studies, which I will be discussing in the following chapters, are worthless. It would do this not to celebrate those correlation studies exclusively, or to claim that they are superior to any other study design, but simply to consider a broader range of evidence.

A general appreciation for wholism would encourage our research specialists to be more diligent and effective in their communication, not only with other specialists in their fields, but also with those in other relevant fields. Again, I do not think this is a dangerous suggestion. Reductionism encourages compartmentalization; each field or subfield is considered distinct, each with its own journals, conferences, and exclusive jargon. If these characteristics did not prohibit the useful interchange of ideas, they would not be an issue. But they do, and they are. And as a result, we create intellectual silos and more confusion. For example, even within nutritional science faculties, there is great confusion about the meaning of the word "nutrition." Each reductionist subset of "nutrition" has its own way of defining it; I can cite several instances over many years when faculty in the same academic department, who prided themselves on scholarship, suggested that we needed to get together and hash out the true meaning of the word!

By embracing the vast interconnection of research topics, wholism does not exclusively seek clear-cut, black-and-white answers. Rather, wholism encourages the humble acceptance of our own continually evolving ignorance—the idea that each new research finding contributes to a greater understanding of the world (or sheds light on previous misunderstanding) and how we might more effectively thrive within it. Wholism strives toward a more complete understanding of the vast integrative systems that characterize our bodies, our environments, our societies, and the like, but highlights that we can only ever strive, and never reach a hard-and-fast final answer. In this striving, wholism does not compromise our standards of evidence. If anything, it demands an even higher standard of evidence than the current one. It does not reject evidence, but demands that we consider the whole body of evidence. It encourages us to use a wide array of study types, and to understand the appropriateness of certain types of studies for certain subjects and the inappropriateness of other study types for other subjects. It encourages us to interpret this wide array of study types not only as isolated and distinct events but also as parts of a larger whole.

Wholism does not reject Hill's useful criteria for the evaluation of epidemiological evidence. On the contrary, it celebrates and bolsters them by adding a new, tenth criterion: breadth.

New Criteria for Reliability of Evidence

Criterion	Explanation
1. Strength	When there exist strong associations (e.g., a ten-fold size of effect versus a two-fold size of effect) . . . they are generally viewed as more reliable.
2. Consistency	When the findings of a hypothesis by different authors and different study designs agree . . .
3. Specificity	When size of effect and significance of a single causal factor is much greater than for other factors . . .
4. Temporality	When the cause precedes the effect . . .
5. Gradient	When the effect increases with the exposure, or "dose" . . .
6. Plausibility	When a hypothetical cause can be explained mechanistically . . .
7. Coherence	When the findings of a study align with other generally known facts . . .
8. Experiment	When carefully designed experimental tests of a hypothesis agree . . .
9. Analogy	When analogies or similarities exist between the observed cause-and-effect relationship and other well-accepted associations . . .
10. Breadth	When an association exists across divisions of age, gender, ethnicity, etc.—when it exists in a broader context . . . it should be viewed as more reliable.

Breadth of effect is especially important in the case of nutritional effects, which I will discuss in greater depth in chapter eight. Breadth asks whether an intervention might be used to treat a fuller range of illness and disease; it asks whether recommendations might apply, at least in part, for everyone, regardless of age, ethnicity, and sex; and crucially, it asks whether an intervention may be capable of both treating *and* preventing disease. In short, this single addition makes a huge difference. Emphasizing breadth of effect results in a profound departure from current pharmacologic treatment protocols, which almost exclusively target the alleviation of individual symptoms on an illness-by-illness basis, and even on a treatment-by-treatment basis within a single illness!

Again, this should not be taken as a repudiation of the original nine criteria. No doubt, Hill's original criteria are very useful. But they also conform to a reductionist model of disease causation. By adding breadth—that is, by refocusing our attention on *the whole*—we correct this issue. Whereas a reductionist assessment of evidence can be misleading and even potentially dangerous, breadth is far more discerning. For example, there may be very compelling evidence indicating a certain diet's ability to promote weight loss, and that evidence could very well satisfy most of the nine old criteria. But what if that diet also had adverse effects on other measures of health? What if it also promoted loss of strength or loss of balance among older adults? What if it only resulted in weight loss for young women, and did not have a similarly beneficial effect for older men? Obviously, we would prefer a diet whose positive effects worked across the board, so why would we not consider the evidence for an intervention in an across-the-board way, too?

The point I'm circling again and again is that good evidence should satisfy the principles of both reductionism and wholism. Though there's an obvious value in knowing how certain mechanisms work and how certain interventions influence those mechanisms, this knowledge must also be meaningful within a broader context. If a piece of "good" evidence cannot help to clarify the true nature of the whole, then it doesn't matter how well it delineates a specific mechanism. If we are committed to truly useful science, then we must keep our eyes on the prize—the *whole* prize—and not let ourselves slip into a self-congratulatory cycle of highly specialized quests for trivia that the public can neither understand nor use.

Or, to put it more mildly, we need balance.

FOR THE SAKE OF HEALTH

I have chosen to introduce reductionism and wholism in a fairly general, abstract sense because I believe that reductionism's limits and wholism's benefits apply to all fields of science (and beyond). But make no mistake: the exclusive dominance of reductionism is far more harmful in certain fields of science than in others. At the top of this list, I put the health sciences.

The vast majority of individuals involved in the health sciences are good people, but their system is letting them, and us, down. In medicine, the dominance of reductionism translates to an ever-sharpening focus on individual diseases and their specific treatments. It is regularly assumed that each and every disease has a specific cure. At every turn in the system we are met with a highly skilled specialist: one to research the individual mechanisms of the disease, another to develop the drug, another to perform the surgery, and even one to labor over who will pay the bill. But we are all paying a greater price, because Nature cannot be tricked into the specialist's box. Nor can health crises that afflict the whole body and arise as a result of numerous causes interacting dynamically, even symphonically. Each and every "side" effect of our current preferred treatments (including drugs, supplements, and surgery) testifies to the insufficiency of our reductionist practice and to the wholistic nature of health and disease. Our "treatment" of preventable diseases like cancer is characterized by reacting to symptoms rather than proactively addressing their causes; by dangerous, unnatural, pharmacological "solutions" with shockingly poor success rates and many unintended problems of their own; and by exorbitant costs for both individual patients and society as a whole.

We should not be surprised, therefore, that our health care system is always playing catch-up. Reductionist specialization is perfectly suited to the study of disease as we have come to define disease. Health—which is not merely the absence of disease, but actually the complete opposite of disease—is too large a subject for any one specialty. So long as the time and energy of virtually every medical professional is tied up in the reactive treatment of disease, the mantra of our medical system will never be health promotion. Even within individual specialties, disease *treatment* occupies so much of our time and energy that we fail to address disease *prevention*. Changing this would require a broader understanding of health and disease than our current system can manage.

Again, this is not a critique of the trusted specialists who make up our "health care" system, as individuals. I do not fear them, I fear *for* them. I fear for their impossible task of promoting health well past the point of disease's takeover. Specialization is a phenomenal tool, but it cannot be our only tool.

Where, then, does that leave us? And what about nutrition? Informed experts in the field of nutrition *should* be better equipped to discuss the control of disease, since food is linked far more naturally to health, disease, prevention, and treatment than any pill or invasive procedure. When you eat health-promoting foods, you feel healthy, and vice versa; preventing unhealthy outcomes becomes a mere matter of careful observation and appropriate action. This may seem like something of an oversimplification when considering larger populations, but my larger point is this: whereas drugs and procedures *react*, food *provokes*. Even if we aren't mindful and deliberate about provoking healthful outcomes, we have not escaped food's grip. More likely we have simply forgotten food's natural powers and are mindlessly letting it string us toward disease and death.

Nutrition, then, as a provocative but natural science, offers a unique opportunity to radically challenge and depart from the disease-maintenance system that currently burdens our society. Perhaps this is even its principal role. That nutrition, *as it currently exists,* has not issued this challenge on a wide scale is a condemnation of the broader medical system, in addition to nutrition scientists themselves. Mirroring the rest of science, the field of nutrition has adopted its own reactive, reductionist, highly specialized approach—an approach that does not line up with how nutrition really works. In fact, the very concept of "reductionist nutrition" is an oxymoron. Sadly, though, this is what the field has become, and in so becoming, nutrition's potential to prevent and treat many of our most dreaded diseases has been reduced. By dividing nutrition into its smallest components, and by studying those components simplistically and in isolation, nutrition has been cheapened to the point of uselessness.

What we need now is a radical overhaul of reductionist nutrition.

CHAPTER EIGHT

THE LIMITS OF REDUCTIONIST NUTRITION

People are fed by the food industry, which pays no attention to health, and are treated by the health industry, which pays no attention to food.
—Wendell Berry

We must not be afraid to address the failure of nutrition—the systemic misapprehension that dominates the field—in an honest and full way. This must include not only the challenges discussed in Part II, which considers the dysfunction *within* nutrition, but also the broader set of challenges introduced in chapter seven. These are challenges *beyond* nutrition—challenges that ensnare nutrition. They indicate a wider web of dysfunction, the dysfunction of all science, characterized by the exclusive dominance of reductionism. As in a healthy system or a healthy body, this dysfunction is not simply the sum of all our mistakes: the whole-ness of our failure far exceeds the sum of its parts.

You may recall from my analysis of the history reviewed in Part I that nutrition has long been marginalized and ignored in the traditional research and treatment of cancer and other metabolic diseases, and that conventional treatment protocols were able to consolidate under a few powerful institu-tions, which continue to dominate research and treatment today. Naturally, I believe this marginalization is crucial to understanding where we are now, but I'd like to move past it for a moment. Easy though it may be to paint researchers who study the connection between nutrition and cancer as vic-tims of a corrupt, exclusive system, that narrative doesn't do enough to propel us forward. It is a factual critique, but misses a very important point: there's more than enough blame to go around, and scientists in nutrition are not exempt.

After all, if the story were only that of a corrupt, exclusive system, we wouldn't expect to see so many peer-reviewed papers cataloged on the National Library of Medicine's PubMed website under the search terms "Diet and Cancer" and "Nutrition and Cancer"; there were over 55,000 as of the beginning of 2020. Given that number, shouldn't we have more answers to (if not a consensus on) the big questions, such as whether a clear link between cancer and nutrition exists? Even more fundamentally, why has the nutrition research establishment thus far failed to reach a consensus on the healthiest diet? I see this failure not as proof of individual error, but as proof of a broken concept, proof of pandemic misunderstanding, proof that our questions about nutrition (guided by reductionist science) have been damned at their roots.

As one of that crowd of nutrition researchers, I am embarrassed that in spite of the impressive quantity of research conducted during the last fifty to seventy-five years, many nutrition scientists continue to squabble over its details. Of the nearly 55,000 peer-reviewed papers I mentioned, the overwhelming majority assume reductionist nutrition as a framework of analysis. The consequences of this are significant. Unlike in certain other fields of science, where reductionism is used, for example, to design and test pharmacologic agents intended for target-specific receptor sites, the exclu-sive dominance of reductionism in nutrition does far more harm than good.

We are dealing with Nature, which harmonizes, through metabolism, our incredibly varied nutritional needs. This means we need to be very careful in our interpretation of reductionist research findings. To describe or interpret Nature's processes through reductionism alone is insufficient and often dangerous.

We have not been very careful so far. Rather, we have fallen deep into the well of reductionist thinking. This is why the ability of food to maintain health and prevent disease is described almost exclusively in reference to individual nutrients. Although information about individual nutrients can be helpful in certain cases, this approach lends itself to dangerous tunnel vision. Even if we accept the complexity of whole foods on an intellectual level, reductionism has become so normalized that experimental and exploratory research on the independent activities of nutrients often blatantly ignores that complexity. We proceed to study individual nutrients as if their activities in isolation are the same as their activities in whole foods, when in reality there are often many significant differences between the two (including, in the case of isolated nutrients delivered via supplements, unanticipated harm).

This approach—focusing solely on nutrients acting "independently" within food—has been the core mode of studying food and health for many decades. Dietary guidelines on food consumption from the early 1940s until 2002 were based on the recommended daily allowances (RDAs) of individual nutrients. In 2002, dietary recommendations were expanded to include a range of "safe" intake levels for individual nutrients. Likewise, food labels and health claims have long emphasized the importance of individual nutrients. It's even seeped into public knowledge and shaped our valuation of specific foods. We are told that the beta carotene in carrots is good for eyesight, that the vitamin C in oranges prevents colds, that cow's milk provides vitamin D and calcium to make strong bones and teeth. Growing up, I was urged to *go on, eat the liver! It's a great source of iron. You don't want to become anemic, do you?* And if you're like most people, the food that comes to mind when you hear the word "potassium" is bananas. Meanwhile, the same logic applies in the other direction. You might have heard that eating too much spinach can decrease calcium absorption due to its oxalate content, or that the carbs in potatoes increase obesity and diabetes risk, or that the estrogen in soy causes breast cancer. You might have heard that fatty nuts increase the risk for heart disease; though in the case of nuts, there's a good chance you've heard the opposite, too.

Maybe it's time to add bewilderment to the long list of epidemics that plague us?

You might be thinking that these nutrition details don't seem especially threatening. But the stories we tell ourselves are critically important. They shape our beliefs and behaviors. Think about your own life. If you constantly tell yourself that you're not good enough, what is the result? Does it breed confidence, self-esteem, and enlightenment? Of course not. The stories that pervade our society and shape our beliefs and behavior act in the same way. When virtually all the stories we tell ourselves about "healthy nutrition" are splintered, contradictory, and missing context, how can we expect a healthy result? The Old English root of the word *health* is derived from the Old English word *hælth*, meaning "whole," and yet our notion of healthy eating is tied only to a jumbled mess of fragmented food facts, some true and some not.

And so, as they now stand, our concepts of nutrition and health are incompatible. By focusing only on reductionist nutrition, we are deliberately ignoring the wholeness of health, and these concepts will continue to remain incompatible so long as our nutrition fails to acknowledge and serve the wholeness of health. Can you imagine prescribing daily servings of *tomatoes*—or worse, lycopene supplements—to a patient who has just suffered a stroke? Of course, no doctor would rely on giving such advice, and only a desperate patient would take that recommendation with a smile, for they will suspect (and rightly so) that they aren't being told the whole story. Perhaps this is also why today's nutritionists don't get the same respect as seemingly sophisticated surgeons and drug developers. All three provide incomplete solutions that do not fully address the underlying cause of disease, but at least the surgeon or drug developer's solutions feel more definite, technologically impressive, and productive.

The recommendation of a "complete dietary lifestyle overhaul" is of course far less passive than a prescription of tomatoes, but this is not what today's nutritionists are trained to recommend. Clinical dietitians and nutritionists today are "educated" by the Academy of Nutrition and Dietetics (AND), and let me tell you—they do *not* advocate for wholistic nutrition. I have been invited to give keynote presentations to their national convention three times, most recently in 2008 in Chicago. On that occasion, the registration bag provided to all participants proudly displayed AND's corporate partners, including drug companies (GlaxoSmithKline), junk food and beverage companies (Coca-Cola, PepsiCo), and dairy interests (National Dairy Council). After sharing my contrary views that year, I have never been invited back.

Within such a controlled environment, today's nutritionists are not fulfilling the full potential of their field. Not because they are bad people, but because the system is ill. They offer bland, easy, nonthreatening advice, suggesting that we give low-fat yogurt a chance, pat on the back included; some even peddle supplements. How could they not? Examples like these are precisely what comprise reductionist nutrition. And neither did yesterday's nutritionists research complete dietary lifestyle overhauls (or not in the main, at least). In the small number of cases in which researchers did seek more comprehensive evidence for nutrition's role in diseases such as cancer and heart disease,[1] they faced considerable pushback.

With that past and this present in mind, is it any wonder that the future of nutrition looks impotent alongside its peers? Consider the following examples:

- Of the approximately 130 medical specialties recognized in the United States, nutrition is not one of them.
- Nutrition is virtually untaught in medical school.
- It is nearly impossible for physicians to receive reimbursement for nutrition counseling.
- Despite an impressive combination of international epidemiological studies and laboratory studies that have indicated a potential role for nutrition in treating cancer, nutritional therapy continues to be neglected as a treatment protocol, or even as a possibility.
- The most recent estimate for total NIH investment in nutrition research[2] is $1.9 billion in 2020, to be spent on 4,500 individual research grants, slightly more than 1 percent of the agency's total budget. I am familiar with the claim that additional nutrition research funding occurs in the specific disease categories of NIH,

but to the extent that this may be nominally true, the money is for investigations involving specific nutrients as pharmaceuticals (nutraceuticals) and non-nutrient pill and procedure remedies.*

- Let's put this in perspective: a rough but very conservative estimate for annual pharmaceutical R&D is $71.4 billion, almost forty times greater. (This estimate is also substantially below the industry's estimate, while the $1.9 billion attributed to nutrition includes a great deal of research not directed toward fundamental investigations of nutritional function, and certainly not toward investigations of wholistic nutrition; given this, it would be easy to suggest a ratio closer to 100:1.)

But again, nutrition professionals are not exempt from blame for this exclusion and underappreciation. In our commitment to reductionism, we in the field of nutrition have zoomed in so far that we can no longer see our own value. We should not be surprised that no one else can either.

AN ILLUSTRATION OF REDUCTIONIST NUTRITION

When I was teaching introductory biochemistry in the 1960s, I taught what is now a well-known pathway of biochemical reactions within cells, a sequence of "end to end" reaction pathways beginning with a sugar molecule (glucose) formed in plants and packed with energy from the sun through the process of photosynthesis. Looks like a fairly complex system, right?

---

* My experience comes from twice giving private presentations to National Cancer Institute director's staff on nutrition priorities and funding.

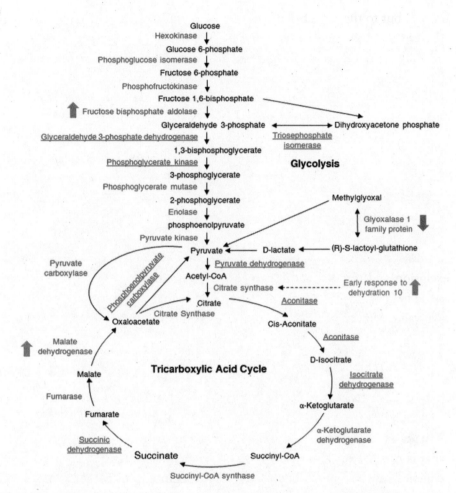

Image by Alqurashi, M., Gehring, C., and Marondedze, C., from DOI: 10.3390/ ijms17060852, reproduced under Creative Commons License (CC BY 4.0).

Perhaps it does, but complexity is relative. In this newer chart, you can see that over the last fifty years, many reactions have been discovered and added to our understanding of this pathway:

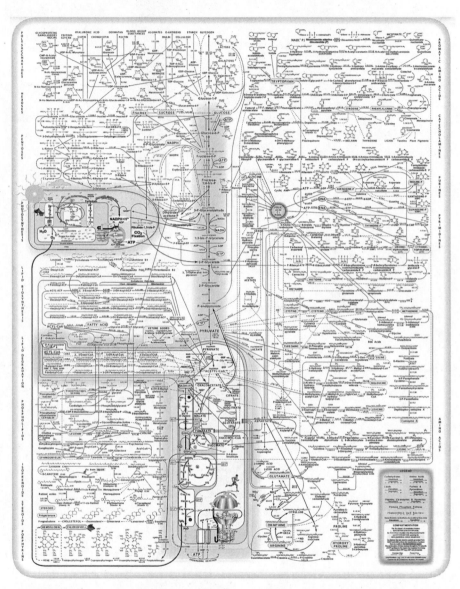

Metabolic map prepared by Dr. Donald Nicholson on behalf of the International Union of Biochemistry and Molecular Biology, reproduced with permission.

And this chart, busy as it is, still only barely scratches the surface, displaying only a minuscule fraction of the total reaction network. It is a poor illustration of the infinite complexity of metabolism—of Nature—not only because it is incomplete, but because it will always be incomplete. Finitude has always had an impossible time painting infinitude. Poets know this obstacle well; too many scientists pretend it doesn't exist.

For our purposes, though, the illustration is clear enough: it is an orgy of information attesting to unknowability. It suggests to me that we will never fully understand the mechanistic and thermodynamic relationship of food, health, and disease. That we are staring into an abyss and that we always have been. And that, in our investigations of nutrition, we have fused the practice of arrogance with the spirit of naïveté; to presume that Nature is chartable, we must have thought highly of ourselves and poorly of Her. But that's *okay*. What's important, now that we know how little we know, is that we take a step back now and look at the big picture—that we identify those foods that are natural for our consumption, the foods that optimize this infinitely complex process, and that we have the wisdom to get out of our own way.

The alternative, continuing down the path of reductionist nutrition, is simply unacceptable.

TOMAYTO, TOMAHTO

Let's look briefly at three examples of how reductionism has not only failed to clarify nutrition, but in fact has obstructed its clarity, beginning with our tendency to rank foods by their nutrient densities. This practice is a perfect example of both how far nutrition has strayed from its potential and how firmly it has latched on to reductionist methods, two sides of the same coin. It's also a great example because it has become such a mainstream practice. Nearly everyone is at least somewhat familiar with the concept of nutrient density. Conventional wisdom has, in this case, become the spitting image of common idiocy.

A few years ago, cow's milk would have topped most lists of nutrient-dense foods, although kale is now a far more common winner. Granted, the order of such a list depends on which nutrients you measure and what biological target is being affected. I could easily make the case for a number of different foods as the most nutrient dense, based on which nutrient is chosen for the index and which of its multiple functions are used to define its overall value. This wiggle room allows for considerable "creative interpretation," to put it nicely. But the problem with this system of ranking foods is not only that it lends itself to cherry-picking (or udder-tugging), but also that the measurements themselves are highly variable and not conducive to practical recommendations.

To illustrate both of these points, consider the contents of three nutrients for seven vegetables generally thought of as similar in nutritional value (all numbers, pulled from the USDA's "FoodData Central" database,[3] the most highly regarded nutrient database, have been rounded to two significant figures):

Chart 1. Nutrient Variability for Seven Sample Foods

Vitamin C, mg/100 g	Raw	Cooked, Boiled	% Change
Kale	93	18	–81
Broccoli	89	65	–27
Peppers, sweet, green	80	74	–8
Turnip greens	60	27	–55
Peas	40	14	–65
Swiss chard	30	18	–40
Spinach	28	10	–64

Beta carotene, mcg/100g			
Turnip greens	7000	0	—
Spinach	5600	6300	+12
Swiss chard	3600	3600	0
Kale	2900	1700	–41
Peas	450	470	+4
Broccoli	360	930	+158
Peppers, sweet, green	210	260	+24

Magnesium, mg/100g			
Swiss chard	81	86	+6
Spinach	79	87	+10
Kale	33	25	−24
Peas	33	39	+18
Turnip greens	31	22	−29
Broccoli	21	21	0
Peppers, sweet, green	10	10	0

Rank order	Vitamin C	Beta Carotene	Magnesium
Kale	1	4	3
Peppers, sweet, green	3	7	7
Peas	5	5	4
Turnip greens	4	1	5
Swiss chard	6	3	1
Spinach	7	2	2
Broccoli	2	6	6

My purpose for presenting these data is to show how varied are the nutrient contents of foods, an observation almost never shared with, or recognized by, the public. When we compare the contents of three specific nutrients in these seven vegetables—a water-soluble vitamin (vitamin C), a fat-soluble vitamin (beta carotene), and a mineral (magnesium)—we see their nutrient contents vary widely. (This is true of these foods in their raw form, but particularly when they are boiled. Boiling food generally decreases nutrient contents, but not always.) As to which food is the "most nutrient dense," this depends entirely on which nutrients are considered, as seen in the rankings. Similar findings could be shown for many other food–nutrient combinations as well. Try making your own list of foods; look up their nutrient contents and you will see the same thing.

What these foods all share, then, is an exceptional nutrient variability. And remember, these seven foods are already relatively similar, at least when compared to foods in other food groups.

I'm unsure how the public is supposed to leverage this information, given the amount of nutrient variation. Should I feel better knowing that my raw broccoli has 3.2 times more vitamin C than your raw spinach, even though the latter has 15.6 times more beta carotene and 3.8 times more magnesium? These differences are huge, and yet they still only tell a sliver of the story. In particular, what about other nutrients in these foods, and what about the effects of their interactions? Can any of us say which food is healthier? And how do we extrapolate dietary advice from these numbers, or make health predictions? Might I get one-third as many colds from my diet of raw broccoli, when compared to someone on a raw spinach diet? What is the trade-off? On the beta carotene front (where spinach ranks more highly than broccoli), am I sacrificing potential gains in eyesight?

It would be ludicrous to use nutrient density rankings as a means to compare foods and infer specific health differences, not only because of the convoluted logic that it would require, but also because it falls way beyond the scope of even the most sophisticated consumer. It would take a team of supercomputers to determine the optimal diet based on such rankings, and even then, it would require far more information than we currently have. Who at your local grocery store has the time and energy to parse out this information?

So who is benefiting from this jungle of nutrient content information, if not us and our fellow shoppers, and what do they gain? The most obvious beneficiaries, from my perspective, are food processing and marketing specialists, groups that make up a growing, disturbing breed of capitalist specialists. In their world, profit and growth take precedence over our bodily, societal, and environmental health. This is not to say that health and profit are wholly incompatible, just that health, and especially long-term health, falls lower on these food processors' list of priorities. Health is still vitally important to many of them, but not in the way you would like: more often than not, they commodify and package health not out of a shared human interest, but as a shortcut to greater profit and growth. It doesn't take a nutritional biochemist to see this commodification in action. Walk the aisles of one of your local "health food" stores and you will see shelves stocked mostly with processed nonfoods starved of health but featuring a variety of clever labels touting recent health claims. Where these manufacturers succeed is in selling an *image* of health.

I came to know this very well when I served for three years, at the behest of the National Academy of Sciences (NAS), as the principal witness during the Federal Trade Commission hearings on health claims. The main claim concerned a company that wanted to take advantage of our 1982 NAS report advocating increased consumption of vegetables, fruits, and whole grains by making health claims about their supplements that the evidence showed applied only to whole foods. (This was also part of an intense campaign to revise food and drug regulations, thus opening the door for developing a nutrient supplement industry.) They were denied, but in the long run, their and others' efforts succeeded in launching the vitamin supplement industry as we know it.

The concept of nutrient density in particular, as a stand-in for health, lends itself to many marketing ploys. Sometimes they involve perfectly good foods, as in the case of so-called superfoods. These are foods the market tells us to consume due to their exceptional health qualities, often related to one nutrient or another. For the most part, they *are* good foods—I enjoy kale, pomegranates, and many of the other foods labeled as such—but our portrayal of them is not without consequences. For one thing, an emphasis on superfoods doesn't do nearly enough to provoke broad dietary lifestyle changes to the standard American diet. In fact, it may have the opposite effect, giving consumers a false sense of security and self-congratulation. The sad fact is that most Americans' diets require a far more drastic change than the incorporation of, say, açaí berries, delicious though they may be, and it makes little sense to single them out unless you're basing a business on them.

To that point, many of the foods touted as super also come with a super-high price tag, which reinforces the average consumer's false impression that health is only for the wealthy. As health has become increasingly commodified, higher price has also come to imply higher health value. That healthy eating will break your budget is one of the most common, dangerous myths about healthy eating, and the sooner we upend that narrative, the better. While headlines trumpeting maca powder's miraculous benefits may be interesting, and may serve an elite class, our attention would be much better directed toward the "peasant foods" that save lives: garbanzo beans, rolled oats, sweet potatoes, and so forth. Unfortunately, those foods don't glow with the same luster, in part *because* they are so common, and the exclusivity of specialty foods is part and parcel of their appeal. This is Marketing 101, selling not just the image of health but also a smug feeling of superiority.

Food processing and marketing specialists benefit from nutrient density rankings in other ways, too, some of which are far more insidious than the sales of healthy foods. Perhaps the most important of these is also the most fundamental: nutrient rankings reinforce the individual nutrient's place at the center of nutrition. By giving primacy to the nutrient, rather than the whole foods and dietary patterns that contain them, we invite all kinds of shenanigans. In a world where individual nutrients are given precedence, the consumer doesn't bat an eyelid when these nutrients are extracted and bottled as supplements (a potentially dangerous practice we'll discuss more below), or when unhealthy foods are "fortified" to give the pretense of health (a practice that may boost certain foods' nutrient contents but not necessarily ensure a healthy food overall). Producers don't bat an eyelid either, but rather lick their lips.

FURTHER VARIABILITY IN NUTRIENT CONTENT

Up until this point, the issues I have been discussing take it on faith that the nutrient content of foods has been accurately measured, and that the greater the accuracy, the greater the return on health. To take the topic of nutrient density seriously, and to dispute its usefulness *on its own grounds*, I have allowed these two assumptions. But we should back up now and test these assumptions, for when it comes to a broken system, nothing can be taken on faith.

First of all, the USDA's laboratory measures of nutrient content are subject to the same standard variation associated with repeated measurements in any other instance. When measuring the nutrient content in a single sample, even the most conservative estimate assumes *some* variation from the mean, perhaps ranging from 5 to 20 percent when all modifying variables are considered. When you expand beyond a single sample—say, one particular piece of broccoli—to consider the nutrient contents of a larger group of samples, it results in a more reliable estimate of the mean. But it turns out that a pot of boiling water isn't the only thing capable of radically changing the nutrient content of our favorite foods. Other than the variation arising from analyzing even the same sample multiple times, even greater variation results from several other factors: when during the season the plant is harvested, where in the environment it is harvested, how it is processed, and how much time passes before consumption. Each of these factors will contribute additional nutrient variation among different samples of the same food; taken together, they compound our uncertainty of nutrient content to a startling degree. The bottom line is this: at the time of consumption, we can only roughly approximate the nutrient content of the food we are eating.

What's striking is that the USDA database doesn't mention this variability. In fact, it seems to go out of its way to imply greater precision. For example, the beta carotene content of grape leaves is listed in the database as 16,194.00 micrograms per 100 grams—seven significant figures! Since we know that these numbers are given to variation anyway, surely it would make more sense to round off to three significant digits, at most, as in 16,200? I can only guess at the motives of this nutrient database's creators. Perhaps they would like to lend an air of greater accuracy. What I do know is that highly precise numbers do not mean more reliable science. It's often said that liars provide far more details than necessary, to compensate for the uncertainty and mistrust they anticipate in their audience; I wonder if the same might be true here.

And if you think that's bad, things become far trickier once a nutrient, either in food or pill form, is swallowed and left to wend its way through the body. On the journey from your lips to its functional site, the nutrient must pass through many layers of screening and adjustment: digestion, intestinal absorption, serum transport, cellular entry, intracellular metabolism, and finally distribution in the body. Each of these steps is carefully managed by your body's systems, which regulate both how much of the nutrient is allowed to pass and how quickly it does so. Differences in transfer rates from one stage to the next are often major; extensive evidence shows that the amount passing through each stage can easily vary by 30 percent. During intestinal absorption, this variation can reach 90 percent.[4] In short, the relationship between the amount of nutrient consumed and the amount arriving at its functional sites after passing through so many stages of compounding uncertainty is incalculable.* To put it simply, Nature has the tools to do what

* According to the calculations of my friend Damon Demas, PhD, a freelance mathematician, if 1280 mcg of a nutrient were consumed and 50 percent were to pass through each of six checkpoints on its journey to its functional site, an average of only 20 mcg would reach

she wants, easily adjusting how much of a nutrient is brought to its site of action. She controls a wide-open game, essentially saying to us, "Leave it to me. I will drive how I want, however fast is appropriate, to wherever we need to go. You only need to bring the right kind of supplies and I will do the rest. Oh yeah, and don't toss in a lot of stuff that I have to spend my energy cleaning up!"

We've already seen how complex Nature can be and how much it can contribute to nutrient variation, even within the same species of plant. But the crucial and often forgotten fact is that humans are also Nature. Yes, no matter how much we like to pretend otherwise, *we* are Nature. Like the rest of Nature, our bodies are far more intricately balanced than we give them credit for. They determine not only how much of a nutrient passes from stage to stage, and how quickly, but also how much of the nutrient is metabolized—changed into new products, metabolites, that actually carry out the nutrient's function in the body—as well as when and where those metabolites will be used. Each metabolite may act, with varying degrees of potency, on different tissue targets. Some nutrient metabolites may be as much as a thousand times more or less active than their parent nutrient.

Even if it were possible, through reductionist science, to measure all the reaction rates and learn all the metabolites a single nutrient produces, that information would still be useless, because these rates change. They change in response to the presence of other nutrients and they change over time—*even within a single nanosecond*. And these processes are occurring, all the time, in each and every one of our tens of trillions of cells. The body's process for integrating the nutrients we consume is a highly dynamic system of reactions, occurring at many levels in the body, constantly working to establish optimum function.

All of this uncertainty may seem bewildering—if you're unable to comprehend the immense complexity of the body, you're in good company—but it need not be. What's important is that we don't trick ourselves into thinking we know more than we do. Within such an awesome system, reductionist

---

its final destination. But assuming a reasonably normal variation in "pass-through" at each checkpoint, Nature would deliver either less than 8.6 mcg or more than 31.4 mcg more than 30 percent of the time.

biochemistry can only take us so far. We must eventually draw on other virtues, like humility. I say this as someone who has devoted my life to biological chemistry: we must let go of our need to know *everything*. We must observe more intelligently, and respect what we have already learned. Once we do so, the uncertainty will no longer result in a sense of hopelessness. Rather, it will inform a greater realization: that the human body is a highly intelligent force of Nature. That the body will take care of itself if you provide the necessary resources and tend to its external environment. We have sacrificed far too much time and effort on a fool's errand—arming some of our brightest, hungriest minds with only their microscopes and spectrophotometers and asking them to see the universe, to convey its depth not only accurately but also comprehensively. But knowing how to care for the body requires that we move beyond an exclusive focus on reductionist nutrition—beyond obsessing over the amounts of individual nutrients found in individual foods.

THE CALORIE DEBATE

A second example of reductionist nutrition can be found in our outsized focus on calories. This topic has permeated the community of food and health for many years, and if it is not addressed it will continue to cause confusion.

At the risk of oversimplifying the debate, we must consider two points of view. The first contends that the effect of diet on health is primarily due to the *amount* of food consumed; the second argues instead that the *type* of food consumed is more important.

I first became aware of this debate when the McGovern Committee of the US Senate suggested, in 1976 and 1977, decreasing average dietary fat from about 35 to 40 percent of total calories to 30 percent of total calories, in a specific effort to control the occurrence of heart disease. Despite being very moderate, that recommendation threatened several industries, including the livestock industry. The counterargument thus arose that it was not the type of food consumed, but rather the total amount of food, also described as the number of calories, that impacted health—and thus, consuming 40 percent of calories from fat was not necessarily going to cause heart disease, so long as the total number of calories was not excessive. Simply count calories and eat what you want.

Many questioned this calorie-in, calorie-out proposal because a high-fiber, plant-based diet (in other words, eating a certain type of food) has been shown to help manage how calories are used—for example, how excess calories are disposed of through additional exercise and/or through burning off those calories as they are used to keep the body warm.[5] Some have even said that we could eat more and weigh less, so long as we ate the right kinds of food.[6,7]

To this day, scientists have not reached a consensus, and the issue remains a public debate, because there is some truth to both points of view. There is no doubt that body weight may be controlled by carefully monitoring calorie intake, regardless of the content of one's diet, coupled with regular exercise to increase calorie expenditure.[8] Moreover, it is also possible to gain weight on even a WFPB diet, as some have discovered, through a combination of excess calories and inadequate exercise.[8] I am not aware of any professionally published, peer-reviewed research studies that have satisfactorily reconciled these observations in a way that satisfies all.

This much, however, is clear: by focusing primarily on calories, we miss the greater context of health. It may be possible to reach a desired weight by focusing mostly on calories, regardless of type of diet, but this does not ensure health, especially in the long term. Focusing on body weight as a measure of health is also reductionist. Although being overweight or obese is associated with many health problems, that does not mean weight loss is the be-all and end-all for improving health. There are many ways to lose weight by unhealthful means, including crystal meth. Diets that promote weight loss but do not support overall health are not inherently healthy diets, appealing though they may be to our superficial, image-obsessed society.

That aside, the clear takeaway from these decades of debates is that focusing heavily on calories has done little to clarify the role of nutrition in promoting health. In fact, it has by and large distracted the public's attention from nutrition's most profound powers, which have less to do with weight control than they do with the control and reversal of deadly diseases.

LITTLE NUTRIENTS
MAKE A BIG INDUSTRY

It should be clearer by now that reductionist nutrition is an impoverished shell that offers very little help in correcting our current disease maintenance system. Nutrition scientists' stubborn loyalty to the reductionist model has had a number of consequences, two of which (an inaccurate understanding of nutrient density and a distracting debate on calories) I have discussed. A third example is the development and growth of the nutrient supplement industry.

Here I mainly refer to supplements of individual vitamins and minerals, and combinations thereof, which received a huge boost in 1982 when the NAS published its report on diet, nutrition, and cancer.[1] Compared with today, the vitamin and mineral supplement industry was relatively small and disorganized, although public interest in consuming these nutrients was considerable. After the discovery of vitamins and minerals during the 1920s and '30s,[9] the market size of the supplement industry grew from $700,000 in 1925 to $32 million in 1935, and to $83 million in 1940. It is now projected to be $216.3 billion in 2026.[10] Talk about finding Fort Knox down a rabbit hole!

Throughout the mid-twentieth century, considerable discussion took place on the legal and regulatory control of these supplements, to ensure they would be marketed safely. The chief regulatory question seemed to be whether these substances should be classified as foods or drugs, or neither, while the chief medical question concerned their efficacy and safety. At the time of our 1982 NAS report, the most significant regulation on vitamin supplements was the recently enacted 1976 Proxmire Amendment, which overturned the existing FDA regulation that supplements must adhere to an upper "safe" limit of 150 percent of the recommended daily allowance of a vitamin. By this time, rising public interest was translating into considerable political pressure.

It was because of that interest that we chose in our 1982 NAS report to address the issue of what role (if any) that isolated nutrients as supplements might have in helping to control cancer. We explicitly stated in our executive summary that our recommended goals concerned whole foods as the source of nutrition, not nutrient supplements.[1] I remember how clearly we emphasized in the executive summary that "these recommendations apply only to foods as sources of nutrients—not to dietary supplements of individual nutrients."

I also remember how, in spite of this, the supplement industry tried hard to secure a laxer regulatory environment for marketing their products and advancing their health claims.[11,12] A relatively small, loosely associated group of "health" companies saw this period of time as an opportunity to "go big"—to double down on the supplement products the public was clamoring for. So in the years immediately following the 1982 NAS report, the NAS subsequently requested that the Federal Trade Commission (FTC) hold administrative court hearings on the health claims being made in favor of nutrient supplementation. At the behest of the NAS,* I spent three years as the principal witness questioning those claims.[13] What I testified to then and what I stand by now, based on the most current evidence, is that the nutrient supplement industry's health claims are vastly insupportable. Several studies have proven supplements' ineffectiveness,[14-16] and indeed even signaled that nutrient supplementation may sometimes be *dangerous*. But that didn't seem to matter then, and it doesn't seem to matter now. Those FTC hearings were little more than a speed bump, and the industry has been flying ever since. Its sales pitch is far too easy to swallow and not challenged frequently enough by those who should know better. Eat what you like, avoid what you don't, and plug the gaps with magic pills. Not sure where your gaps are? No problem, we'll find them for you. In a time when nearly all our greatest killers—heart disease, cancer, diabetes, and the like—are the result of *excess*, this industry insists that we must somehow be *deficient*.† A ridiculous inversion, clearly, but at least you don't have to eat Brussels sprouts.

Eventually, in 1994, the supplement industry's efforts culminated in another highly significant amendment to the FDA regulations, called the Dietary Supplement Health and Education Act (DSHEA), now recognized

---

* I received no personal remuneration.

† Of course, when one's diet comprises mostly non–whole foods, certain deficiencies may result, but this absolutely does not justify the use of supplements; rather, it makes the case for WFPB nutrition even stronger. By doubling down on supplements, we are only reinforcing the bad habits that cause deficiency.

by the industry as the most important piece of food and drug legislation of the last century. It widened the doorway for developing an endless number of dietary supplements and the beginnings of a massive market. By 1994 the industry had already expanded greatly since the 1982 NAS report, reporting $4 billion in sales, 4,000 products, and a customer base that included about half of the adult population. But the 1994 amendment paved the way for even more growth. Now, twenty-six years later, 77 percent of Americans report that they consume dietary supplements, with a projected global market of $230 billion by 2027!

Since those early-'80s FTC hearings, the scientific research community has conducted numerous NIH-funded human intervention trials to determine whether nutrient supplements, either individually or in combination, might work. The findings have been in line with the assertions in the NAS report—which is to say, discouraging. Often nutritional supplements had little or no effect on disease risk, and in some cases they found that the supplements *increased* it.[17] One of the earliest studies that focused on a presumption of single-nutrient effects involved the antioxidant beta carotene, a metabolite of vitamin A.* It had been shown that smokers consuming a *diet* high in beta carotene experienced substantially lower lung cancer risk.[18] At about the same time, a second study of 1,954 male smokers showed that the incidence of lung cancer decreased by seven-fold across four categories of beta carotene consumption. This remarkable association of greater beta carotene consumption with less lung cancer was particularly impressive for the subset of subjects who had smoked at least thirty years.[19] This is obviously not to say that smokers should puff away, so long as they consume beta-carotene-rich foods, but these findings were truly extraordinary and sparked great interest from the supplement industry. Subsequently, an eight-year study was planned to determine whether beta carotene *supplements* might have a similar effect on another group of smokers—but the researchers had to pull the plug early when cancer incidence among those in the supplement group shot up from 36 percent to 59 percent.[14]

---

* When vitamin A was discovered, it was (and still is) called retinol. However, a nutrient is defined as something that must be consumed because our bodies cannot produce it. Retinol is, by definition, not a vitamin nor a nutrient because we make it in the liver, using the beta carotene that we consume. Thus the real vitamin is (plant-made) beta carotene, not retinol.

There are many other examples of studies in which individual nutrients, isolated from food, have produced an effect opposite from their presumed behavior in food—so many, in fact, that it seems to me that nutrition researchers should by now have gotten the clue. Moreover, further summaries (meta-analyses) of individual nutrient trials have confirmed supplements' inability to confer significant health benefits.[16,20] Several well-respected news outlets have since echoed these findings. In 2013, WebMD headlined, "Experts: Don't Waste Your Money on Multivitamins."[21] A similar Science-Daily headline in 2018 read, "Most Popular Vitamin and Mineral Supplements Provide No Health Benefit, Study Finds."[22]

Surely these intervention trials and the generally consistent message about supplements' ineffectiveness should have sounded the death knell for this phony industry a long time ago. So, what gives? Sadly, the supplement industry's greatest lifeline is the public's yearning for health. The sicker we become, the more we seek shortcuts to health; the more we seek shortcuts, the more vulnerable we are to industry's claims, particularly when their recommendations are palatable and require very little effort on our part. A recent vitamin supplement industry report[23] spoke very directly to this point: "Healthy Forecast: An Aging Population and Growing Health Concern Will Supplement Growth." That "healthy" forecast projects that the industry's 2018 annual revenue of $31 billion will grow at a rate of 1.9 percent, and pegs total industry employment at 36,404 spread across 1,383 businesses. In the report, the industry congratulates itself for meeting a "growing interest in wellness and nutrition among mainstream consumers." Meanwhile, other projections show that mainstream consumers will become even more interested in supplements over the coming years. According to projections from Grand View Research,[24] a US-based market research and consulting company, the size of the dietary supplements market (including botanicals, vitamins, minerals, amino acids, and enzymes) will reach $230 billion by 2027, as previously mentioned. A large part of their projection relies on the continued rapid rise of obesity rates in developed economies, and on the fast-food sales and sedentary lifestyles in "emerging economies including India and China," which they anticipate leading to an "increase in the prevalence of cardiovascular disorders, diabetes, and obesity."

These projections provide further proof of what should by now be obvious: a booming quick-fix industry is not only an effect of increasing sickness, but also one of its greatest fans. If we are going to banish nutrition-related, preventable diseases, we will have to face its profiteers as well. The most important thing, however, is that we learn to face our own complacency. According to the same Grand View Research projection, higher-income groups of the future are increasingly "expected to perceive . . . dietary supplements as the alternatives to prescribed drugs."

The contrast between the research on nutrition supplements and the mostly false claims encouraging their continued use, as well as the public's attitude toward them, could not be clearer. Our advertising and beliefs about supplements directly contradict both nearly four decades of research and a number of professional research panels that have reported on the association between food-based nutrition and cancer[1] as well as related diseases.[25–27] The messages coming out of this research have been generally hopeful. What we eat *does* make a difference. The research does not, however, support the same for supplementation of isolated nutrients. That practice is nothing but the ugly offspring of a ménage à trois starring reductionism, marketability, and the downward trajectory of our society's health.

Reductionist supplementation, like the examples of the previous two sections—the practice of ranking foods by their nutrient densities and the debates surrounding calories—distract public and professional attention away from how nutrition might be used to prevent and even treat disease, and create a great deal of unnecessary confusion. All three of these examples have undermined the potential in the field of nutrition. If we aren't more careful and if we do not consider alternatives to reductionist nutrition, then the future may not be long lived.

THE ALTERNATIVE: WHOLISTIC NUTRITION

None of this is to say that there is no place for reductionism in nutrition science; as I stressed several times in chapter seven, the focus of my critique is not on reductionism itself but on its exclusive dominance. Until balance is restored, the science of nutrition will remain as I have described it thus far in this chapter: an elaborate system for collecting conflicting information that neither medical professionals nor the public know how to apply.

To restore that balance, and maximize the potential of this science, I propose a *newly defined, wholistic* nutrition.

Wholistic nutrition demands that nutrient-specific evidence and recommendations enter the debate if and only if they enrich our understanding of the greater context. There are certainly cases in which such nutrient-specific evidence and recommendations can enrich our understanding of that greater context, but we must be vigilant and never lose sight of their purpose: the promotion of whole food consumption and whole-body health, *as supported by the greater scientific context,* which ultimately breeds a healthier society, species, and planet. Likewise, insights about specific foods may have a place in this discussion, as with research into so-called superfoods, but we need to be far more discerning in the kinds of questions we ask about specific foods and even food groups, far more critical when assessing the relevancy of supporting evidence, and far more responsible in the way we report on that evidence. To reiterate a point made in chapter seven, wholism does not reject evidence, but rather demands a higher standard of evidence. It demands that we consider the whole body of evidence. Trapped in the tunnel vision of reductionism, it's easy to disorient consumers' valuation of spinach due to the isolated effect of oxalate on calcium absorption. However, taking care to understand and communicate the whole body of evidence around the health-promoting effects of spinach leads us to a much more logical end—say, perhaps, a salad.

To take that point a step further: not only does a wholistic perspective on nutrition improve our approach to nutrient- and food-specific recommendations, it also demands a less simplistic assessment of how those nutrients and foods act in the body. Wholism acknowledges, and even celebrates, the highly integrative manner by which nutrients operate. Wholism concerns itself less with individual mechanisms than with how countless mechanisms work together toward the same end, which is health. Moreover, it concerns itself with the broad consequences of nutrition's effects on health and disease. It concerns itself, in this sense, with *breadth* just as much as *depth*.

When we adopt a wholistic perspective on nutrition and health, two key lessons emerge. First, by its emphasis on the wholeness of health, nutrition, and food, wholism is by definition opposed to the consumption of unnatural food fragments. This includes not only supplements but also highly processed products like refined sugars, oils, and other drug-like substances that are *manufactured* to keep you wanting more, despite the suffering they inflict on your body, your community, and the planet. The whole body of evidence, as well as public perception, is in general agreement on the unhealthiness of these products. Dieters of all shapes and sizes mostly concur that soda is not a healthy beverage, though I'm sure we could find some who disagree. (Apparently there are also groups of people who still believe the Earth is flat!) This consensus is hardly surprising. There's a reason we call it "junk food." Even the most far gone Apple Jacks addict can intuit that the food on their spoon is nothing but a broken replacement for the whole subsistence provided by Nature in foods like apples. Second, based on the kind of wide and diverse body of evidence emphasized by wholism, the healthiest dietary lifestyle is one that is exclusively plant based. Together, these two lessons recommend a diet that has been the center of my professional work for the past three decades: a whole food, plant-based (WFPB) diet.

I introduced this diet in the earliest pages of this book as the focal point of a great deal of controversy, which I have since tried to delineate. I have described this controversy as it relates to disease care, as it relates to animal protein and other nutrition myths, and now as it relates to science and evidence. As I have unfolded each layer of this controversy, I have drawn your attention to bits and pieces of the supporting evidence in favor of this dietary lifestyle. But it is important now to focus more pointedly and fully on that evidence; if it could not withstand that scrutiny, then its controversy would hardly be worth discussing.

CHAPTER NINE

A CASE STUDY
OF WHOLISTIC
SCIENCE

What lies beyond us and what lies before us are tiny
matters compared to what lies within us.
—Ralph Waldo Emerson

Trying to research the WFPB diet through scientific protocols typically used for reductionist research is like trying to weigh a horse using only a tape measure; there is a fundamental incompatibility between the subject of study and the means by which we study it. A WFPB diet simply cannot be tested using that "gold standard" double-blind, randomized controlled trial, for a number of obvious, logistical reasons. Though it may be possible to test certain, individual food items in this way—for example, it may be possible to manufacture a placebo flaxseed meal capsule filled with the same texture or flavor as real flaxseed meal—it is impossible to do the same with an entire diet, especially one that emphasizes whole foods.

We must therefore consider a broader array of evidence for WFPB nutrition. We must look at a wider range of research studies—including studies that satisfy reductionism and its standards of "good" research, and studies that don't—and we must interpret them, within a larger context, as parts of a whole. Moreover, this evidence should be held to the highest possible standard: evidence in favor of a WFPB diet should be overwhelming. This is not to say that the evidence should be absolute. Just as the evidence indicting cigarettes in the case of lung cancer is not absolute, evidence in favor of a particular diet will never be absolute. Nevertheless, no rational person would dispute the overwhelming weight of evidence against cigarettes and smoke them in the meantime, and I believe we can reach a similar conclusion as it pertains to diet. This is a very old idea: in the absence of absolute evidence, one should take the cautious approach and adopt the protocol for which there is the best available evidence, especially when there is no evidence that contradicts it.

This wholistic approach is what I have been working on from mid-career onward, if not always with full awareness of how to define it. Throughout that process, I have relied on vast amounts of published evidence from both contemporary research and studies published before my lifetime. For my own part, I spent many years earlier in my career caught in the ruts of reductionism, and I learned a lot of valuable information from that research. I asked simple questions and conducted simple experiments, mostly in the laboratory, from 1965 to 1997. By studying single causes, effects, and explanatory mechanisms, I was able to pursue relatively provocative questions without upsetting the applecart too much. Most of these questions concerned diet and nutrition's effect on cancer. But in the confinement and isolation of conventional academic practice, none of that research proved as valuable as it does now, in full context. Neither was it as provocative in any of its fragments. It was only when I synthesized these findings in a broader context, within what I now recognize as the natural order of things, that the apples started flying.

THE EVIDENCE SUPPORTING
A WFPB DIET

The entire body of evidence favoring a WFPB diet could not possibly fit into one book, much less one chapter. Other books, including *The China Study*, have surveyed some of this evidence more completely than I will here, but even those cannot capture the continuous evolution of this field. To keep this section succinct and not sacrifice other valuable elements of this book, I have made many choices regarding evidence. What follows, then, is a sampling of what I consider the most relevant and potent.

Keep in mind that these pieces of evidence do not exist in a vacuum. They are best assessed in relation to one another. I issue this word of caution just as much to those in the plant-based community as to anyone else. In my experience, proponents of plant-based diets are no more immune to reductionism than anyone else. Many capitulate to specific interests, whether in the sale of nutrient supplements or the pursuit of personal fame and fortune, and it would be a grave mistake to ignore our own fallibility in this regard. Thus, while dividing these pieces of evidence makes for easier reading, we must always remember that it is only by integrating them that we attain a more profound understanding of nutrition and its impact on human health.

CORRELATION STUDIES

Reductionist researchers in the nutrition field almost universally disagree with using observational, correlation studies in support of, well, anything, because correlation studies do not prove causation. This mantra is one of the first things scientists are taught, a lesson that I myself taught as a university professor for many years. And it is a perfectly valid lesson *if* we are searching for single causes of single effects—say, for example, if we're seeking a single, specific nutrient that promotes ovarian cancer—as in reductionist nutrition. In that case, it's easy to say, "Well, saturated fat appears *correlated* with ovarian cancer, but it may not necessarily *promote* ovarian cancer. The correlation could mean nothing; ovarian cancer could also be caused by x, y, or z." The major flaw in this critique, however, is that it assumes ovarian cancer can be attributed to a single cause in the first place.

On the other hand, if we assume a wholistic definition of nutrition, in which a multitude of nutrients act in synchronicity, and we interpret correlation studies in reference to broad dietary patterns rather than specific nutrients, we gain far more insight. By the wholistic definition of nutrition, we would presume from such a correlation neither that "saturated fat causes ovarian cancer," nor that "$x, y,$ or z could also cause ovarian cancer," but instead consider how a broad array of nutrients work in simultaneous combination to promote several cancers. By reframing the concept of cancer causation as multifactorial, our interpretation of correlation studies *ceases to indict specific nutrients out of context*. Rather, it considers specific nutrient–disease associations only as a means to illuminate the greater dietary context. However, lest it be forgotten: reframing the wholistic argument as akin to multifactorial causation can also be limited if it only focuses on the factors that we consume and if it assumes that these factors act independently when present in tissue. I believe that a more complete description must also include the interplay of factors during metabolism. In statistical analysis of cause and effect, this is referred to as second- and third-order variance.

For example, in all of the following correlation studies, I use animal protein, or its surrogate,* as the independent variable. But I do *not* do this to suggest that animal protein *alone* causes various cancers, as a reductionist interpretation implies. I use animal protein because, as we've discussed, its consumption is a phenomenal determinant of *broad dietary patterns*. In a whole food context, one cannot consume animal protein without consuming animal foods, and unlike saturated fat, animal protein cannot be removed from animal foods. It is thus used here as an indicator of larger dietary trends. In particular, since eating and becoming full are effectively a zero-sum game, eating more animal protein also indicates eating fewer plants. It is my view, based on available research, that both of these patterns, which are inextricably linked, contribute to the development of degenerative disease.

---

* The term *surrogate* here refers to a stand-in, or statistically significant correlate. Using highly correlated surrogates emphasizes that multiple variables can contribute to the development of disease and health.

Charts 1 to 10 on pages 212 through 216 display correlations between diet and disease rates (either mortality or incidence, depending on the chart) for different countries. All charts are reproductions of data as they were published, and all charts show a straight-line association of disease rate (or its indicator) with consumption of animal protein (or its surrogate).*

Chart 1 is derived from a publication on the associations of total, saturated, and unsaturated fat consumption with breast cancer mortality.[1] I relabeled these fat intakes as "animal protein intake" after getting permission back in 1989 from the author, Professor Ken Carroll, a highly accomplished diet and cancer researcher of that period, who agreed that my interpretation was novel and correct. Though not indicated here, the study showed no association of breast cancer mortality with plant protein. I first presented this reinterpretation that year to a National Academy of Sciences committee, of which Carroll was a member, that was preparing a major report on diet and disease.[2] I published that interpretation[3] many years later, in 2017, in reference to heart disease because (1) the consumption of animal fat is highly correlated with the consumption of animal protein ($r = 0.94$)[4] and (2) I had learned of animal studies conducted during the early 1900s suggesting that animal protein experimentally increases early heart disease[5] more than cholesterol itself.

Chart 2 was published in 2005 by a different group of authors.[6] It records breast cancer *incidence* rather than mortality and cites meat intake as the independent variable rather than animal protein intake (which also includes dairy and eggs). Despite these differences, its findings are essentially the same. The observed link between meat consumption and breast cancer incidence strongly reinforces the breast cancer mortality results from chart 1 and suggests that any amount of increase in meat consumption is theoretically associated with increased breast cancer risk.

Chart 3 shows an association of uterine cancer incidence with total fat consumption[4] in a different set of countries. Just as with chart 1, total fat is highly correlated with animal protein, making it an effective surrogate. Also,

---

* All straight lines (linear regressions) except for one (in chart 8) were approximated based on an equal number of data points appearing on both sides of the line. Note that the lines are straight and that they intercept the *x–y* origin for animal protein, suggesting that a diet without animal protein reduces the rate of cancer incidence and mortality to zero.

similar to chart 2, chart 3 shows a strong correlation between diet and a cancer of the reproductive system.

Chart 4 shows the association of colon cancer incidence with meat consumption in women, and chart 5 the association of renal cancer incidence with animal protein consumption in men.[4]

Chart 6 shows the association of prostate cancer mortality with nonfat milk, another good surrogate; because the fat has been removed, nonfat milk is composed primarily of animal protein. Again, it suggests that diets containing more animal protein suffer an increased incidence of cancer, in this case prostate cancer.

Moving on to diseases other than cancer, chart 7 (from nearly fifty years ago!) shows a linear association between cholesterol intake and heart disease in twenty-four countries.[7] It shows that as cholesterol intake decreases, so too does heart disease risk. Cholesterol intake is an excellent surrogate for animal protein intake because cholesterol is found exclusively in animal foods.

Chart 8, published in 1959,[8] displays the logarithmic association of heart disease mortality with animal protein (for twenty countries).

Last, charts 9 and 10 show the association of bone fracture rates, which indicate osteoporosis—a chronic degenerative disease often wrongfully assumed to be the inevitable result of aging—with, respectively, calcium and animal protein intakes, both of which are primarily provided by dairy products. These plots are comparable to chart 6 for nonfat milk and prostate cancer.

By shifting the focus toward animal protein and its surrogates *as indices of broader dietary patterns* rather than *sole causes of disease*, and by interpreting these graphs in a more integrative way (challenging the assumed separateness of these diseases and looking at the often-ignored dietary relationship that underlies all of them), we profoundly challenge the way that research of this kind is usually interpreted. I understand that, in the intepretation I'm about to offer, I'm going out on a limb, as far as the traditional scientific community is concerned, but it is intentional. After all, I am more concerned with presenting this information practically but meaningfully and reliably to the public, where I believe its impact will be greatest. With that understood, here are a few summary points:

- All graphs are unaltered original data that suggest the same conclusion: excluding animal protein consumption correlates with little or no disease.
- All of these animal protein–related correlations should be interpreted as a combination of the direct effects of animal protein plus the indirect effects caused by decreased consumption of whole plant-based foods. I use the term *animal protein* rather than *inverse-plant-based foods* (also acceptable) in order to emphasize the long-time, cult-like desire of many people to consume meat and other animal products as a means of good nutrition.
- The breadth of this animal protein effect on various diseases (several cancers, heart disease, osteoporosis) is impressive.[9]
- *No correlation study has ever shown the opposite relationship*; that is, no studies have associated high protein consumption with the decreased incidence or mortality of these diseases. This suggests that these correlations are highly reliable.
- This reliability is further strengthened by these findings' remarkable consistency. These results represent the work of many authors, across decades, in several types of disease.
- The likelihood that such consistency might be attributed to chance, especially when coupled with the absence of any contradictory studies, is unbelievably low.

To return to where I began, I would grant once again that correlation does not equal causation in a reductionist model, when hypothesizing that a single agent causes a single disease. But, importantly, nutrition does not belong in a reductionist model. By broadening our scope to consider disease formation as multifactorial, and considering only factors that are representative of a broader dietary pattern, as in the case of animal protein, we virtually erase the potential for confounding variables. Furthermore, I find it extremely unlikely that any of these findings could be attributed to non-nutritional factors, as these chronic diseases not only have been linked with nutrition for a long time but also have been linked to nutrition more convincingly than to any other lifestyle or environmental factor (e.g., sedentary lifestyle, environmental toxins, etc.).

Chart 1: Breast Cancer Mortality

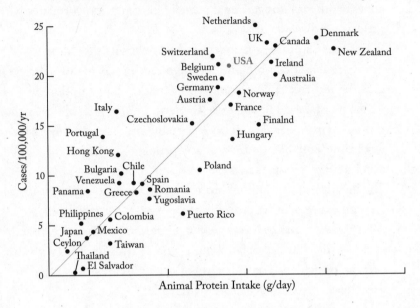

Chart 2: Breast Cancer Incidence

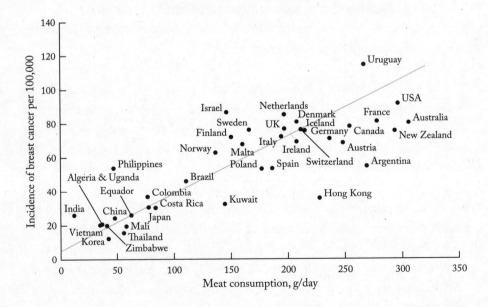

Chart 3: Uterine Cancer Incidence

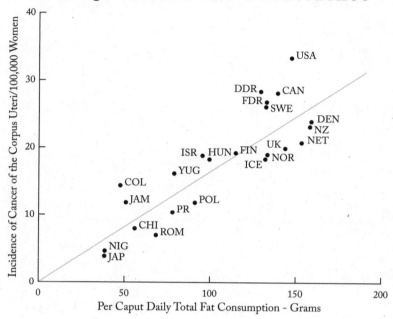

Chart 4: Colon Cancer Incidence

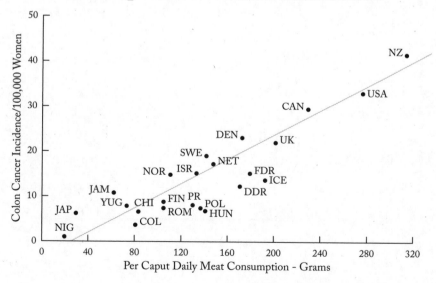

Chart 5: Renal Cancer Incidence

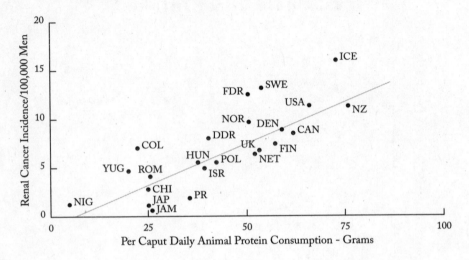

Chart 6: Prostate Cancer Mortality

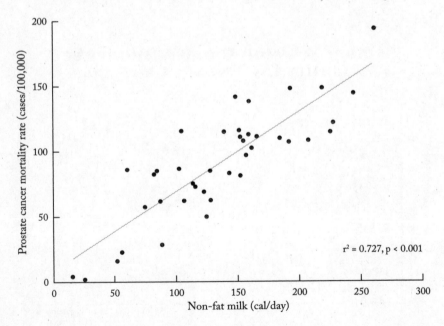

Chart 7: Coronary Heart Disease vs. Cholesterol Intake

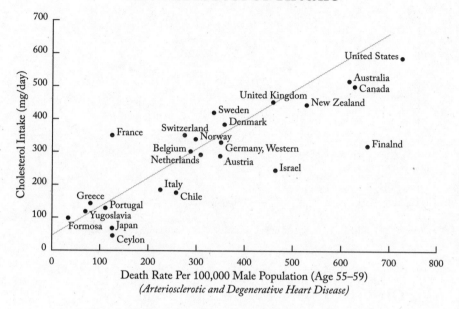

Death Rate Per 100,000 Male Population (Age 55–59)
(Arteriosclerotic and Degenerative Heart Disease)

Chart 8: Coronary Heart Disease Mortality for Twenty Countries

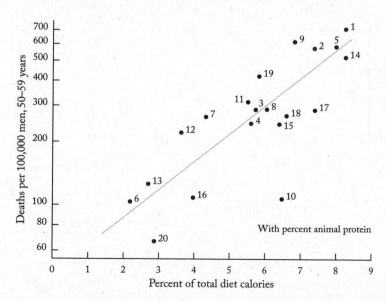

Percent of total diet calories

Chart 9: Hip Fractures and Calcium

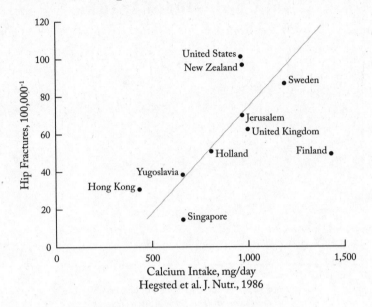

Calcium Intake, mg/day
Hegsted et al. J. Nutr., 1986

Chart 10: Fractures and Animal Protein

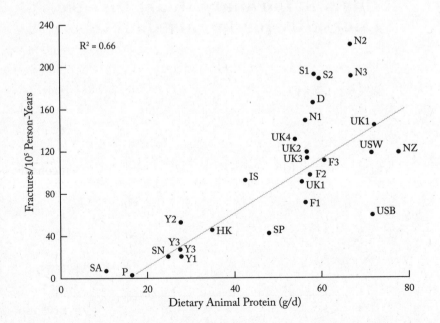

Dietary Animal Protein (g/d)

Lest I be too glib here on the "driver" status I've assigned to animal-based protein, it is theoretically possible that processed foods, which vary widely in nutrient composition, could be a driver, at least to some extent, in combination with animal protein. But the nutritional effects and nutrient content of processed foods are so hugely variable that it would be virtually impossible to determine which component of these foods and which affected target would account for this generalized effect, and whether such a component would or even could function as a driver. Most importantly, it would be almost impossible to identify explanatory mechanisms amid so broad a category of food. Though reductionist on their own, such explanatory mechanisms (which I discuss below) do provide strong support for wholistic evidence (e.g., the correlation studies mentioned above).

Last, though more limited than the evidence linking an animal protein–rich diet to heart disease and cancers of the breast, uterus, colon, kidney, and prostate (charts 1–6), similar findings also exist for cancers of the mouth, pharynx, larynx, nasopharynx, esophagus, lung, stomach, pancreas, liver, endometrium, and cervix, as summarized in a very large review of diet and cancer[10] and in a single study showing a large effect of nutrition on melanoma.[11]

Evidence from these correlation studies is compelling on its own. If there existed complementary evidence of biological plausibility—that is, evidence showing *how* animal foods produce this effect—then the case would be even more convincing. We will get to that shortly. But first, we should consider another highly impressive type of evidence that supports the benefits of a WFPB diet.

INTERVENTION STUDIES

I have already described why a randomized controlled trial, often considered the gold standard of all research studies, simply does not work for testing a whole food diet. Everyone knows which group they are in, and further, it is almost impossible to randomly assign subjects to their respective groups. Can you imagine people faithfully consuming a diet that, for a variety of personal reasons, they do not like? And even more unlikely, can you imagine such a study lasting for an extended period of time, as is required to assess a diet's long-term effects? In the nutrition field, this type of intervention is ideal for testing drugs and drug-like supplements, but its usefulness ends there. We must therefore look at other types of intervention research studies. When we do so, particularly in the case of heart disease intervention studies, we find that the effectiveness of WFPB nutrition in preventing and treating heart disease is unrivaled.

The study on diet that has most closely adhered to a reductionist model, randomly assigning patients to treatment or control groups, was conducted from 1946 to 1958.[12,13] You may recall from that study's brief introduction in chapter one that the researcher, Lester Morrison, was a cardiologist who received patient referrals from primary care doctors and alternately assigned a hundred successive patients (average age of sixty) reliably diagnosed with heart disease to one of two diets. The first was a high-cholesterol diet, which included 200 to 1,800 mg cholesterol per day, and the second was a low-fat, low-calorie diet, which included 20 to 25 grams per day of total fat, making up 15 percent of 1,500 total calories, and only 50 to 70 milligrams of cholesterol per day. The first is more typical of the American diet, whereas the second is comparable to what some today might refer to as a "flexitarian" diet: mostly vegetarian, but not as intensive as a WFPB diet. Results from the experimental, low-fat group were impressive: all fifty of the high-cholesterol patients died within the study's twelve years, whereas 38 percent of the low-cholesterol, low-fat patients survived. This suggests that any movement along the spectrum toward a WFPB diet, when compared to the standard American diet—relatively high in fat and animal-based foods—may be beneficial.

Nevertheless, despite its impressive findings and the estimable reputations of its funding source (the American Medical Association) and publisher (the *Journal of the American Medical Association*), the study was met with incredulity. According to a recent review of the decades-long debate on cholesterol, fat, and heart disease, some contemporaries considered the research to be a "fluke (or worse)," and one reviewer even complained that the study was not properly randomized (though his enthusiasm for statin medications indicates his bias).[14]

Almost four decades later, Dean Ornish et al.[15] assigned twenty-eight patients to a year-long lifestyle intervention that featured a low-fat, vegetarian diet. Eighty-two percent of those patients reversed disease progression (they showed less stenosis, i.e., less narrowing of the arteries) without using lipid-lowering medication. Blood vessel health continued to improve in the low-fat group for the next four years, whereas a standard, high-fat group saw a continued decline in blood vessel health, as indicated by further narrowing of the arteries. Additionally, the high-fat group suffered *five times more* coronary events during those next four years.

Caldwell Esselstyn et al.[16–18] conducted a similar intervention study at about the same time, allowing lipid-lowering medication as an option. The findings at five[17] and twelve years[16] showed a remarkable decrease and even reversal of coronary heart disease. Mean serum cholesterol levels at twelve years for the eighteen patients on the WFPB-equivalent diet were 145 milligrams per deciliter.[16] Even more impressive, however, is that these patients experienced "no extension of clinical disease, no coronary events and no interventions" in the years following the study. The consistency of these results is astounding, particularly when you consider the patients' history of heart disease. In the eight years prior to the study, the eighteen patients had experienced a total of forty-nine coronary events!

A subsequent study of 198 consecutive patients suffering from "established cardiovascular disease" showed similarly exceptional findings after follow-ups averaging 3.7 years later. All patients attended one five-hour session of professional counseling in plant-based nutrition. For the 89 percent who remained compliant, only one case of stroke was reported—a remarkable recurrence rate of only 0.6 percent! According to detailed lab tests, the "adverse event rate was at most 10%," again very impressive compared to those in the noncompliant group, 62 percent of whom experienced recurrent events[16] (this was an unusually high rate compared to the expected rate of about 25–30 percent).

Along with the correlation studies displayed in charts 7 and 8 of the previous section, these intervention studies indicate a profound link between WFPB nutrition and both the prevention and treatment of heart disease, which kills about 650,000 Americans every year. The correlation of heart disease with animal protein[8] and the surrogate cholesterol is linear, producing a line that passes through the origin, thus suggesting that *any* consumption of animal protein begins to increase disease risk—a lifetime effect. But these intervention studies also demonstrate the powerful short-term effect of WFPB nutrition. Not only has a WFPB diet been clinically shown to arrest and reverse the progression of our greatest killer—*something demonstrated by no other diet, pill, or procedure*—it has done so in only a matter of months.

This combination of long- and short-term effects is more than encouraging. It meets several of Hill's criteria, introduced in chapter seven: *strength*, *consistency*, *gradient*, and the newly added *breadth*. Given the multitude of studies that have confirmed plant-based foods' ability to minimize risk of heart disease and other diseases, and given that eating more animal-protein-based food aligns with eating less whole plant-based food,* *coherence* can also be added to the list.

LABORATORY EXPERIMENTS

In addition to the more wholistic correlation studies mentioned above, the principal evidence supporting a WFPB diet's effect on cancer comes from, yes, reductionist experimental research studies. These two types of studies complement each other fabulously: lab experiments add depth and reliablity to the correlation studies by helping to explain the association between animal protein and cancer on a biological level. They are the smoking gun, the answer to the question, "*How* could meat consumption contribute to cancer development?" In more technical terms, they satisfy three more of Hill's criteria: *gradient, plausibility*, and *experimental testing*.

My involvement in this kind of research began in the mid-1960s at Virginia Tech, before continuing at Cornell for more than two decades (three when considering further evaluation). During those early years at Virginia Tech—while working on the US State Department–funded program tasked with improving the nutrition of malnourished children in the Philippines, discussed in chapter five. I was studying aflatoxin (AF),[19,20] a potent chemical carcinogen[21,22] found in peanuts (a cheap, versatile source of protein—perfect for our mission of improving childhood nutrition). Around the same time, as I mentioned earlier, I learned of a separate laboratory study on experimental rats in India where rats were exposed to AF, then fed a diet of either 5 or 20 percent of calories from animal protein (specifically casein).[23] The findings of

---

* Please note that food choices approximate a zero-sum game—as you eat more animal-based foods, your remaining caloric capacity shrinks, leaving less space for plant foods.

that study—animals fed the high-protein diet developed substantially more liver cancer—shook my worldview and bent the trajectory of my career.

I sought and received research funding from the NIH to study this question in my laboratory at Virginia Tech, first to confirm the Indian researchers' findings* and then, if possible, to investigate the mechanisms that might explain it. Understanding these mechanisms was especially important given how provocative the findings were; animal protein was, after all, a highly revered nutrient, and we needed to be able to explain not only *what* was happening, but also *how* it was happening. In other words, to return to Hill's criteria, pinpointing the mechanism would show biological *plausibility* and lend credence to the earlier findings.

Before I share my lab's findings, it's important to understand that there are three stages of cancer development: initiation (when mutations are produced), promotion (when cancer cells are replicating themselves), and progression (when cells become more virulent and metastasize into other tissues)—and that each contains within it a vast number of events and reactions. It is precisely in these events and reactions that drug developers would seek a cure, and it was precisely in these events and reactions that we sought to explain the effect of animal protein on cancer.

Stages of Cancer Development

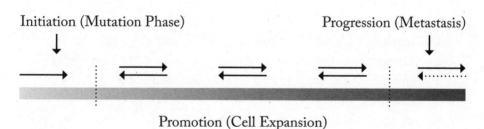

Sets of double arrows indicate the reversibility of the cancer development process.

---

* We did confirm them, finding that cancer development began to increase from a diet of 10 percent animal protein upward, with the first 10 percent being used to support the body's need for protein. Plant-based proteins (e.g., wheat and soy protein) had no such effect on cancer development.[24,25]

Like researchers in the Indian study before us, we initiated cancer using AF, which caused mutations and began the development of liver cancer. We observed that, during *initiation*, AF enters the cell, where it is converted by an enzyme, the mixed function oxidase (MFO), into a highly reactive metabolite, aflatoxin epoxide (AF_{epox}). This metabolite then binds to the DNA (AF-DNA) in liver cells and, if not repaired before the cells divide, becomes a mutation and is passed on to successive generations of cells (*promotion*). Eventually, these cells metastasize: they become aggressive and migrate to new tissues, where they begin the stage of *progression*.

Initiation

$$AF \xrightarrow{\text{Mixed Function Oxidase}} AF_{epox} \xrightarrow{\text{+DNA}} AF\text{-}DNA$$

Promotion

$$AF\text{-}DNA \longrightarrow \text{Precancer Cells} \longrightarrow \text{Tumors}$$

Repaired, 99%+

We investigated ten possible mechanisms during initiation and promotion that we thought might explain the cancer-promoting effect of animal protein. What we found for the initiation phase was that animal protein consumption

1. increases the amount of carcinogen (AF) entering the cell;
2. increases the amount of MFO enzyme available to activate AF;
3. increases the activity of new and old MFO enzyme by altering its 3-D configuration;[26,27]
4. increases the binding of the AF metabolite (AF_{epox}) to DNA, thus increasing its damage;[28,29] and
5. decreases repair of AF-DNA.*

---

* This finding was echoed in the work of Rhonda Bell, from my lab, who also measured the effect of dietary protein on DNA repair with a colleague of mine, Rodney Dietert, and showed that a high-protein diet suppressed DNA repair.

As we discovered more and more deleterious animal protein effects throughout this chain, I began to doubt whether we would ever find a single reaction most responsible for the increase in cancer development. Moreover, each of the mechanisms we discovered during the promotion phase confirmed the same pattern. We found that animal protein

1. decreases the total number of natural killer cells responsible for destroying cancerous cells;
2. decreases voluntary energy expenditure (as measured by the amount of time rats spent on an exercise wheel);[30,31]
3. decreases energy expenditure by brown adipose tissue, which helps maintain body temperature and increases involuntary physical activity (e.g., intestinal motility, heartbeat, breathing);
4. increases a growth hormone that stimulates cancer cell growth; and
5. increases the formation of reactive oxygen molecules that promote cancer development.[32,33]

I'm sure that I could have built an entire career around the pursuit of any one of these mechanisms, and I have no doubt that I could have found more mechanisms in the same reductionist fashion. But eventually, I began to feel that there was a much bigger story here. We had more than enough proof of biological plausibility, in both the initiation and promotion of cancer: the high-animal protein diet increased the activity of eight mechanisms that normally increase cancer growth, and suppressed the activity of two mechanisms that normally prevent cancer.

At first glance, it may seem remarkable that we found no mechanism working in the opposite direction; that is, no mechanism linking a high-protein diet with inhibiting cancer. But when you think about it, this is perhaps the least remarkable finding of all. It seems highly unlikely to me that any such mechanism does exist, for it would seriously disrupt the sequential work of all the others. Why would Nature create such a chaotic and self-contradicting system? (In the area of metabolism, at least, this is unheard of. We do have examples of mechanisms in a sequence, as in a sequence of enzymes, when one mechanism is able to block downstream enzymes—we call them "rate limiting"—but this is not an example of one mechanism contradicting another. In fact, we often learn that it is the down-stream enzyme that sends messages upstream to slow the process. In other words, these mechanisms *work together*, always seeking balance.) Further-more, it would seriously undermine the findings of population studies. As it is, the mechanisms we discovered in our lab experiments only reinforced existing population studies, including the ones mentioned above.

The other big story, from my perspective, was the persistent evidence suggesting that nutrient function is highly integrated, multimechanistic, and downright symphonic—what I now consider the focal point of wholistic nutrition. Just as it makes no sense for Nature to devise a mechanism con-tradicting all others in the progression of cancer, it makes no sense for one mechanism in a sequence to outweigh all others in importance. Likewise, it makes no sense for individual nutrients to act independently, or for any single nutrient to be held more mechanistically accountable than the rest in the formation of health and disease. That is the antithesis of wholism! Ironi-cally, as long as science continues to emphasize separation and reductionism, expressions of wholism appear increasingly self-evident. This is inevitable because wholism is intrinsic to Nature. Even the sequence of mechanisms described above is not as simple and linear as you might imagine. Numerous research reports have since shown how many other single nutrients operate through multiple mechanisms in a highly integrated way—further proof that wholism is the essence of nutrition.

EVIDENCE FOR A COMPLETE WFPB TRANSITION

All of the evidence discussed so far indicates the same thing: we should minimize our consumption of animal foods and increase our consumption of whole plant foods. This is not so different from what you were told as a child: "Eat your veggies!" (It's advice with which virtually everyone in the scientific community already agrees.) The more veggies you eat, the less space you leave for animal foods and non–whole plant foods that are dispropor-tionally weighted down with salt, sugar, and fat. I've singled animal protein out because it is the most relevant indicator or driver of dietary choice. For far too long, it has been singled out in the other direction, as the holiest of holy nutrients. But our reverence for animal protein has outlived its expi-ration date. It's time we retire our interchangeable use of the words *protein* and *meat*, admit that plants provide sufficient protein, and silence that ritual question: "But where do you get your protein?" Soon, I hope to hear a different line of questioning. Where does the average Western diet, with its oxidative stress and chronic inflammation, get its antioxidants? Where does it get its folate, its potassium, and its fiber? Most importantly, where does it get *real* foods, foods that have not been broken and chemically tampered with? We are dying of excess while starving ourselves of Nature's most protective foods.

Still, you may wonder why I suggest a complete removal of animal protein from the diet, rather than, say, an 80 or 95 percent WFPB diet. This is a reasonable question that deserves further consideration. After all, many will argue that the research on this question is insufficient and that not enough studies have compared diets at the healthy end of the spectrum (e.g., WFPB versus WFPB modified to include fish twice per week, etc.). Though I would like to see these, and many others, put to the test, I believe the evidence in support of a cold-turkey approach to cold turkey, and other animal foods, is already very strong (pardon the pun).

For one thing, the correlation studies above show lines of regression passing either through or very close to the origin, where the x-axis and y-axis intersect. This indicates that consuming even small amounts of animal protein may have disease-promoting effects. I don't know about you, but I'd like the diet with virtually no risk, especially when it can be delicious and there are so many other benefits.

Another significant bit of evidence concerns cardiovascular disease and related degenerative diseases, and it comes from my study in rural China, which was a focal point in my first book.[34] There, we found that among 130 villages, heart disease mortality rates* were much lower than for Western countries.† In some Chinese counties, the average number of heart disease deaths was fewer than 1 case per 1,000 death certificates (compared to the nearly 200 cases per 1,000 death certificates in the United States!).[35] Moreover, the rates of heart disease and other Western-type diseases clustered geographically, suggesting that regional dietary patterns played a significant

---

* In people aged thirty-five to sixty-four years.
† Note: Corresponding comparisons with other populations cannot be made because they depend on the age bracket being considered and how it relates to the total population.

role. This disease group (e.g., heart disease, cancers, diabetes, etc.), common to Western countries, was highly correlated* with blood cholesterol, which was, in turn, highly correlated with animal protein consumption.[36] Western-type diseases appeared and began to rise as blood cholesterol rose, within a range of 88 to 165 milligrams per deciliter (mg/dL; mean = 127 mg/dL).[†] That range of blood cholesterol corresponds to *small* amounts of animal protein consumption, about 1 to 12 grams per day. To give some perspective, we in the West tend to consume about 30–65 grams per day of animal protein,[34] with blood cholesterol ranging from 150–300 mg/dL.

In other words, even the most voracious consumers of animal protein in rural China were consuming about 10 percent that of Western countries. Yet *even within that range of minimal consumption*, we observed that animal protein contributed to increased mortality from Western-type diseases. It follows, then, that theoretically the most minimal disease risk would be characterized by a complete absence of foods containing animal-based protein (i.e., a WFPB diet) and a baseline blood cholesterol level of about 90 mg/dL.

If that sounds shockingly low to you, you're not the only one. For decades, the Western blood cholesterol range of 150 to 300 mg/dL has been considered normal. Most authorities today suggest that anything less than 200 mg/dL is "desirable." A graph of one of the most famous studies on heart disease and blood cholesterol, the MRFIT trial of 361,662 men, shows the same association between blood cholesterol and heart disease that we observed in rural Chinese villages. However, it shows this association within a much higher range—one considered "normal" by Western standards.[37] That the Western data shows a still-elevated death rate for older men at a "low" cholesterol level of under 182 mg/dL (about 10 cases per 1,000 deaths), suggests, when considered alongside the Chinese data, that an even lower range of cholesterol is possible. It also reinforces that heart disease can be effectively avoided by dietary and related means. Indeed, one rural county in China reported only one death from heart disease per 265,000 death certificates!

---

* The *p* value was < 0.001, meaning the likelihood that higher blood cholesterol is associated with higher incidence of Western diseases is more than 999 in 1,000.
† The numbers used for this range are county means, meaning some individuals' blood cholesterols were even lower than 88 mg/dL.

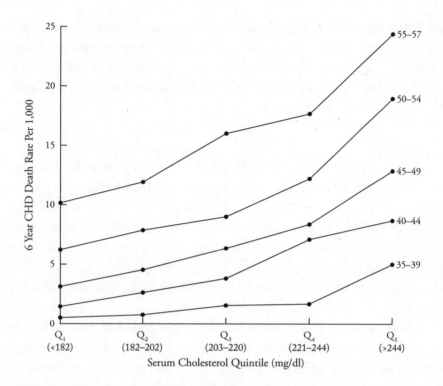

It was with this "normal" range in mind (150–300 mg/dL) that we tested blood cholesterol levels in China and discovered a mean of 127 mg/ dL, which we feared, given our Western mindset, might be dangerously low. And it was within this context that we felt it necessary to retest our samples in different labs and using different methodologies. What we discovered is that these Chinese cholesterol levels were not dangerous at all, unless you believe that reducing one's risk for cardiovascular disease is dangerous. The truth is that our bodies are remarkably adaptable, and the range of what can be considered "normal" is fluid; however, that doesn't mean our society's normal is optimal. When it comes to normal blood cholesterol levels, or "normal" health, we should be very wary of what the medical establishment in Western countries tells us, since it has also accepted chronic, preventable disease as a normal part of aging, even in the young.

There is one final and perhaps most important reason that I advocate for a complete transition to the WFPB diet, and it is that it may be more difficult to adhere to this (or any) dietary lifestyle if one slips back to their old habits from time to time. In other words, a cold-turkey approach may be practiced more easily, for the same reason that smokers are not encouraged to enjoy a cigarette on "cheat days." If it is true that the WFPB diet is the healthiest diet, as I believe the evidence suggests, then there's no good reason to occasionally tempt ourselves.

CONTROVERSIAL SCIENCE IS THE ONLY SCIENCE

Abridged though this presentation of the evidence may be, there you have it: the WFPB diet, as a case study of how we should approach science by both wholistic and reductionist methods. It is controversial in that approach, just as it is controversial for the reasons introduced in the first two sections of this book.

But then, isn't controversy the necessary lifeblood of all science? I am not speaking of the personal attacks of bad or ignorant actors sometimes dragged into the path of science; I am speaking of radical controversy, as I did at the beginning of chapter seven—radical controversy, which disputes the roots of things as they are. The dismissal of the evidence in favor of a WFPB diet, on the grounds that it is controversial, is not an honest engagement with science. The suggestion that this evidence is incomplete is worth debating, but its outright dismissal is proof of a cropped, reductionist approach to science. And I do not believe that approach has served us well thus far.

I don't deny that it would be helpful to have more evidence, and to have a greater diversity of evidence, on a broader spectrum of health and disease. This includes more research studies similar to the ones already discussed, as well as different kinds of research. In the meanwhile, though, we should consider the totality of evidence in favor of a WFPB diet against the totality of evidence in favor of any other dietary lifestyle (including the standard American diet). As long as the opposing evidence remains barren—that is, as long as there are no correlations, interventions, or laboratory experiments that show an effect opposite to the one described above—we would do well to consider the supporting evidence we do have, and to consider it in a wholistic way.

What we should not do is dismiss the overall lesson of that evidence based on lazy critiques of individual pieces of evidence. If all that existed were correlation studies linking chronic disease with animal-based diets, they would be compelling and raise many questions, but they would not necessarily be conclusive. And if all that existed were intervention studies linking WFPB nutrition with the reversal of heart disease (and many other diseases not discussed here), they would be even more compelling and they would raise even more questions, but they would still *not necessarily* be conclusive, just as smoking studies are not 100 percent conclusive. And if all that existed were laboratory experiments showing the mechanisms by which animal protein promotes the growth of cancer, it would be compelling and raise still further questions, but many would rightfully argue that those findings require greater context.

Put all of these pieces together, however, and you see that the totality of evidence in favor of a WFPB diet is broad, diverse, and supported by plentiful context. The next time someone tries to convince you that this evidence is insufficient, you would do well to ask for the dietary lifestyle for which the evidence is *more* sufficient. Ask for both the short- and long-term evidence. Ask for breadth (of disease type, of treatment and prevention, etc.) and ask for depth (has there been both large- and small-scale research, both population and laboratory studies on mechanisms, etc.?). Ask always whether they're selling a product, and whether the health effects of that product have been well documented in both short- and long-term studies. Maybe their evidence will be strong, maybe it will be weak, but you owe it to yourself to ask, and to always interpret that evidence within a broader context.

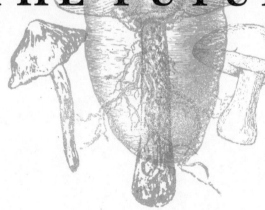

PART IV

LOOKING TO
THE FUTURE

CHAPTER TEN

RECOMMENDATIONS

Peace if possible, truth at all costs.
—Martin Luther

The controversy of the whole food, plant-based (WFPB) diet reveals a number of valuable lessons about how our institutions work. We begin to see how and why institutions authorize certain kinds of science and neglect others, and how and why this affects the funding, publication, and acceptance of future science. The connection between our institutions' attitudes today and the past we remember (or fail to remember) is clear and obvious. But perhaps it would be more accurate to say that these areas of controversy reveal how our institutions *do not* work, when it comes to benefiting the public.

As useful as it is to deconstruct and denounce the current system, we must also think constructively. The challenges we face are complex, too, and so require more than one simple solution. This is why wholism, as an organizing principle to inform our scientific pursuits, is a good first step toward addressing these challenges: it is not merely a rejection of the current status quo, but also an acceptance of something larger and more essential; it does not only question our flawed reductionist practices but offers an engaging, active alternative. By offering alternatives, we don't simply tear systems down, but instead improve them. And shouldn't this be our goal? As broken as many of them are, our institutions are not completely worthless or worthy of total demolition.

Institutions will likely always have some role to play in science and health. They are reasonably good at pulling together information of broad scope (although interpretation of that information may suffer institutional bias, especially when funding sources are taken into consideration). In science, the conferences that professional institutions sponsor can be especially rewarding—provided, of course, that a sufficient breadth of interests is represented. And certain regulatory, legal, and financial objectives can only be achieved by the collective action that institutions facilitate.

The question, then, is not how to obliterate these institutions, but how to flip the script of history and radically transform our systems so that they no longer hinder growth, but rather accelerate it. How can we harness their power for positive change, and redirect their power to empower the people?

#1: ALWAYS QUESTION THE ROLE OF INSTITUTIONS

All institutions that bear power should be subject to the diligence and dissidence of those whom that power affects, including both professionals and laypeople. It doesn't matter whether the institution operates publicly or privately, whether or not it is entangled in our political system, whether it purports to be a nonprofit charity or to feed our children or to educate our students—*whenever* there is a power imbalance between an institution and the people it affects, that institution's role must be justified. People must benefit from the imbalance, however the people may define and concur on what that benefit is.

If, however, an institution cannot justify its power, then its legitimacy should be called into question. If an institution claims to serve the public, but has been proven to sacrifice public service and instead prioritize service to private entities like industry, then its legitimacy should be questioned. There is a vast difference between an institution that pursues its agenda honestly but ineffectively and an institution that serves hidden agendas. One of these may be repaired. The other may be irreparably illegitimate. And if an institution actively discourages or represses the kind of diligence and dissidence I describe here, this is a major red flag that it is the latter.

In the disease-maintenance system of today, virtually all of our institutions must face greater scrutiny and skepticism. Many of them seem determined to undermine whatever claims to legitimacy they once might have held. This does not mean that some of them cannot be improved, but we should at least limit their absolute authority over issues that are well within our own power to control. Here, of course, I am speaking about the benefits of nutrition for health, which should be more widely accessible to everyone. Nutrition, more so than any other biomedical discipline, promotes individual agency. While we cannot very well design our own drugs and perform our own surgeries, we can choose the groceries that we put into our shopping carts. Clarifying the meaning of nutrition is therefore especially important, not only for its ability to prevent and treat disease, but also to restore independence and self-determination. The benefits of eating well are psychological and sociological as well as physiological. And just as clarity in knowledge is crucial to maximizing nutrition's potential, so too is accessibility. Nutrition as a discipline is at its strongest when it remembers that these decisions are *the individual's* to make. They are not Nestlé's choices, or PepsiCo's, or the National Cattlemen's Beef Association's; they do not belong to Cornell University, the American Cancer Society, or any other hallowed institution. Any institution that affects the clarity or accessibility of nutrition—this empowering egalitarian science—should therefore be held to the highest possible standard, and any institution that hinders clarity or limits accessibility deserves to have its legitimacy called into question. In fact, I would argue that this is not only an issue of legitimacy, but also morality.

The tricky question: Who can we count on to question the legitimacy of our hallowed institutions, in the name of public interest?

WILL OTHER INSTITUTIONS PROVIDE BALANCE?

One argument that you might hear, or expect to hear, is that institutions can be more or less trusted to police themselves. After all, each claims to serve the public interest. But in my experience, this is wishful thinking. In fact, I have seen this "policing" firsthand, and it is more often than not the opposite of the kind of policing that one might hope for. Indeed, it is ultimately only another manner by which the status quo is reinforced and minority opinions squashed beyond public awareness.

I have in mind three examples, the first of which concerns two cancer research institutions: the American Institute for Cancer Research (AICR) and the American Cancer Society (ACS). Unlike the much older ACS, mentioned numerous times in earlier chapters, the AICR was founded in 1982 with a very unique focus on supporting research and education on diet, nutrition, and cancer. As the organization's first and only senior science adviser, I was closely involved in its activities during its early years (1983–1987 and 1992–1997), which included coauthoring a trifold pamphlet for 50,000 doctors to summarize the findings of the 1982 National Academy of Sciences (NAS) report on diet and cancer.

As you may expect, the AICR's unique interest in cancer research that integrated nutrition was not without consequences. Once, when giving a presentation to a group of county nutrition extension agents in upstate New York, my host asked me about one of my slides, which mentioned this new nonprofit cancer research society, the AICR. She wanted to know whether I was aware of the organization's allegedly tainted reputation, referring to a "news release" claiming that the AICR was advised by a committee of several physicians who had been prosecuted for criminal malpractice (criminal prosecutions for malpractice are rare in the United States), and that I was the chair of that committee. The assertion was both false and defamatory. Scurrilous lies. I knew about the ACS animosity toward AICR because it had surfaced in a discussion in our NAS committee, when the ACS had asked to partner with our committee in some way in the release of a report. The concern was that the report might paint the ACS as derelict in their responsibility to keep the public informed on this perspective on cancer research. It so happens they were correct in that concern. My suspicion has always been that this libelous misinformation had originated from one of the ACS's executive leaders.

That an organization like the ACS could turn saboteur and work with others to undermine the work of a seemingly complementary organization unfortunately seemed both plausible and likely to me. The ACS viewed the AICR as potential competition for public funding, and they were dogmatically opposed to any mention whatsoever of nutrition as a potential factor in the control of cancer. They viewed their mission as being in support of the medical community.* To return to the original point, if this example is at all indicative of the kind of "oversight" we can expect from competing institutions, then we ought to look for true oversight elsewhere, for this kind of behavior only serves the predetermined interests of the overseer and their industry cronies. It does not disrupt the status quo, but instead intensifies its grip on an unaware public.

As a second example, I later learned of another "policing" group of industry-enthused scientists that met at the O'Hare Hilton Hotel in December 1985 to discuss projects of "great concern" that the American Meat Institute and the National Dairy Council might want to monitor. I have in previous writings referred to this committee as the "Airport Club"[1] because they often met in airport executive lounges. Of the nine projects of concern they initially discussed (later twelve), I had the questionable "honor" of being involved in two. One was our yet unannounced project in China, which had only begun two years earlier, and the other was the AICR. Again, this example speaks to the repugnant encroachment of industry upon science. Who in this example is keeping whom in line?

Yet another example concerns a seventeen-member committee established in 1980 by the American Institute of Nutrition (AIN, now the American Society for Nutrition) to deal with fraudulent diet and nutrition claims in the marketplace. The public relations officer of the AIN's parent federation asked that I serve as a nonvoting, ad hoc member because I was, at the time, the Congressional liaison for the Federation of American Societies for Experimental Biology. The new committee fancied itself as the grand arbiter of nutrition information, a kind of "Supreme Court" for the field that could rule on the legitimacy of all things nutrition related.

---

* Recall the events discussed in chapter two surrounding Frederick Hoffman's role in the founding of the ACS in 1913. His advocacy for taking nutrition seriously was abjectly rejected by the surgeons who took over the organization because of their preference for the local theory of disease.

What followed was demoralizing. Rather than checking and balancing the authority of other institutions, this would-be Supreme Court quickly assumed its own unchallenged authority, deeming itself free to rule on the validity of nutrition claims however it desired. I discerned the reason quickly enough when, at the first meeting in 1980, I saw the chair's proposed news release, which lumped the publication of dietary goals into a longer list of well-known, unacceptable health claims (e.g., health benefits from the use of laetrile, since banned for serious health risks, and pangamic acid, often incorrectly referred to as a vitamin). By associating evidence-based dietary goals with these unproven health claims, they sought to undermine the recent publication of Senator McGovern's much publicized and controversial 1977 report on diet and heart disease, which modestly recommended eating more fruits and vegetables and consuming less fat. Of course, these dietary goals were not at all fraudulent or worthy of this group's attention. When I brought the issue up to my former mentor and committee member sitting next to me, he looked displeased with my reaction, but the news release was withdrawn from the press.

The committee met a second time in 1981 during the annual convention of the Federation of American Societies for Experimental Biology and Medicine. This time, the agenda for our meeting included voting on whether we should recommend to our parent society that our new watchdog committee officially become the intended Supreme Court of nutrition information, hopefully for the whole country. In attendance was Professor Robert Olson, who was serving the last week of his term as president of the AIN. He was obviously there, it seemed to me, to pick up the official recommendation in favor of this committee, now on its way to overall AIN approval and hoping for national prominence.

When it came time for the vote, none of the committee members questioned the recommendation. Nevertheless, I felt I had to speak up. I explained that the committee's activities during the first year had been unimpressive.* We hadn't even established a clear strategy for how we might judge claims of fraud—ostensibly our reason for meeting! In the absence of that clear

---

* These activities included organizing a poorly attended FASEB symposium on fraudulent health claims that was effectively used to advertise a new book by the committee's vice-chair.

strategy, I was concerned the committee would target certain topics without adequate justification, particularly dietary recommendations that went against industry interests.

After I explained these concerns, the chairman stood up and stomped around the end of our long rectangular conference table, where he grabbed the arm of my chair and aggressively shook it. He demanded that I step out of the room so he could have a word with me. I refused, repeating that the committee's activities in the previous year were unimpressive. Just then, an Associated Press reporter knocked on the door to our meeting room. The reporter was obviously there according to previous arrangements to pick up the news release announcing our committee's "positive" decision.

If everything had gone to plan—that is, if the questionable proposal had been ramrodded through without any serious discussion or dissent—AIN president Olson next likely would've presented the good news to the entire AIN membership meeting about to be held. His announcement likely would have been met with the sound of bleated consent, or perhaps only silence. Regardless, the vote was never taken.

I am convinced by these and many other experiences that if we leave our institutions to watch over each other, these kinds of activities will continue. Nobody will demand a higher standard of legitimacy among the powerful. Instead, they will tend toward that old familiar concept, introduced in chapter five: *groupthink*. I'd like to extend that concept to include another wrinkle, by way of political theorist Hannah Arendt. In her 1963 account of Holocaust orchestrator Adolf Eichmann's trial, she coined the famous phrase "the banality of evil" to describe what she witnessed. Her point was not to underplay the evilness of Nazi Germany, but rather to emphasize how evil often appears bland and unassuming. I'd suggest that groupthink, as an institutional reality, operates on a similarly banal level. Sure, there is often drama involved; I know that firsthand. But I also know that groupthink, when pared down to its most essential, doesn't draw as much on the plotlines of Hollywood's psychological thrillers as it does on the mechanical forces of obedience, conformity, and careerism. It thrives on routine. And like any routine, it's easy to fall under its influence without realizing it. If I am skeptical toward institutions' ability to self-repair and keep each other in line, it is due largely to this aspect of human nature—this banal but brutal groupthink.

MEDIA CONTRIBUTIONS

Another argument you may hear is that the media will keep our trusted institutions in line. Again, experience tells me that this is more than a little optimistic, for it ignores how closely many media are entwined with industry. And again, a clear example comes to mind. In the fall of 2016, I was invited by the British Broadcasting Corporation (BBC) to an interview for an upcoming program. I'd long had a favorable impression of the BBC's programs, going all the way back to the mid-'80s when I was on sabbatical leave at Oxford University, and so I was more than happy to agree. Since I had already scheduled a lecture in Chicago at the time of their suggested interview, I used my trip to Chicago to meet them in Cleveland at the home of my friend Caldwell Esselstyn Jr., who was also set to be interviewed for the same program.

It didn't take long to realize I'd been duped. The interviewer, a geneticist from the University of Cambridge by the name of Dr. Giles Yeo, seemed to have already made up his mind about my work and seemed determinedly uninterested in hearing any new perspectives. At the outset of the interview, he admitted to me that he was an "uncompromising carnivore." Most of the two- to three-hour interview was spent riding a golf cart around an orchard near Cleveland, where we discussed some of the research findings from *The China Study*. As we trailed behind a BBC camera crew, their cameras rolling, Dr. Yeo made several comments about how influential my book, *The China Study*, had become and how much of an impact it was having around the world, but I could tell he didn't mean this in a positive way. He insinuated that I should be especially careful with how I spoke to the public, given this success.

Later, I watched Dr. Yeo interview Esselstyn and three of his patients, who discussed their remarkable recoveries from serious disease conditions after switching to a whole food, plant-based diet. Although these patients were very articulate and their stories impressive, it was clear to me that Dr. Yeo was incredulous.

Two months later, when I received an advance copy from the BBC of the finished program, my worries and suspicions were confirmed: it was a hatchet job of the first order, clearly designed to discredit both myself and the evidence supporting a whole food, plant-based diet. The film began by showing the cover of *The China Study*, then proceeded to lump it in with a number of health books that had been widely discredited. One of the authors had even served prison time for his practice on cancer patients! And what of Dr. Esselstyn's interview and his patients' impressive testimonies? Predictably, neither were included in the final film, presumably because they had deviated so extremely from the program's predetermined purpose.

As for Dr. Yeo, his own biases and industry connections speak for themselves. About two months after the interview, he published a paper reflecting his interest in identifying the genetic basis for obesity. The implication here is typical of reductionist research: if we could just identify the *right* gene(s), we might be able to synthesize a drug capable of preventing that genetic expression (never mind considering the food that promotes or prevents obesity!). At the end of the paper, Dr. Yeo acknowledges funding support from the Helmholtz Alliance ICEMED, which consists of "research teams and research centers enhanced by cooperative alliances with Sanofi Aventis Pharmaceuticals and leading international diabetes and obesity research centers at Cambridge . . ." I presume Sanofi, the fifth-largest drug firm in the world, would be more than happy to sell you such a product: a paunch prevention pill.

Naturally, I was concerned about how the program would be received. I knew that anyone familiar with my work would be able to see through this program's transparent aims in a second, but also that most viewers have neither the time nor energy to fact-check every TV program they watch. No matter how slipshod the product may be, many people assume that a credible broadcaster like the BBC simply *knows better*. When I heard that CNN was also scheduled to show the program that week, I knew I had to respond. I quickly emailed my impressions of the film to the BBC director and wrote a short summary and critique for our website. The director was unhappy that I'd posted this article without first consulting him and asked that I also post his own response as well as the responses of Dr. Esselstyn and one of his patients. I obliged.*

* https://nutritionstudies.org/british-broadcasting-corporation-bbc-your-credibility-is
-tarnished/
https://nutritionstudies.org/hidden-british-broadcasting-corporation-bbc
-agenda-dr-yeo-gives-answers/
https://nutritionstudies.org/british-broadcasting-corporation-bbc-credibility-tarnished
-part-2/

A few months after the program aired, I heard from a British gentleman, Gordon MacKenzie, who'd seen the film and was disturbed by its dishonest portrayal of the facts. He contacted the BBC and suggested that they give me an opportunity to respond in some way. When nothing came of that, he complained to the government's media watchdog group, OFCOM, again without success. As of this writing, he persists. Meanwhile, another enterprising English journalist by the name of Klaus Mitchell contacted me. Dr. Yeo had been claiming publicly for some time that he had gotten me to admit that I didn't have evidence to support my claims. Mitchell caught wind of this and subsequently asked to interview Yeo at a conference that he attended. What Yeo didn't realize was that Mitchell was already very familiar with my work and the film's misrepresentation. As expected, Yeo reiterated once again that I had admitted to having inadequate evidence. Mitchell then sent the filmed interview to us and we spliced a few of my own comments in to highlight several points of misrepresentation, faulty premises, and poor science.

I've written a great deal throughout this book about the ways in which useful, evidence-based information on health and nutrition is often silenced. What the BBC affair demonstrates so well is what fills that silence: how sensationalized misinformation is *created*, and how it floods the vacancy left by truth. It shows, in this particular case, the perverse entanglement of a famous media company (BBC), a respected university (Cambridge), a senior government watchdog group (OFCOM), and a multibillion-dollar pharmaceutical giant (Sanofi). These institutions are not collaborating toward the end goal of Truth, or providing checks and balances to one another, but rather consistently tending to mutual interests.

* * *

Who does that leave to question the role of institutions? Honest scientists? Members of the public? People both within and without the systems that organize our lives? Is it naïve of me to place these demands on regular people, with all of our flaws and limitations? And if not the majority of well-meaning people, both within and outside of the systems of power, who can we trust to be diligent and dissident?

I speak as someone who has been deeply involved in the institutions discussed throughout this book. Especially from 1972 to 1997, I worked in many major institutions within the science establishment, while serving on several expert panels, coauthoring reports, and receiving research funding. As a member of the ACS, I once held an unlimited-term membership on their research grants review panel, which recommends which grant applications ACS should fund.* The US government's National Cancer Institute funded about 90 percent of my research (1972–2007), including our nationwide project in rural China (1983–1994).† Furthermore, I served on NCI's Chemical Carcinogenesis study section, presented the Director's Seminar for successive NCI administrations, and successfully organized a petition for a new NCI study section (unfortunately with the suggested word "nutrition" deleted from its title!). I've also long been a professional member of the American Association for Cancer Research (AACR). My research findings have been published in their peer-reviewed journal *Cancer Research* (one of the top cancer research journals).[2-5] Our 896-page China project monograph[6] was also featured on the cover of that journal. Last, I have already described my involvement in the more recent AICR, for which I was the cochair of their sixteen-member international panel that produced a 670-page global perspectives monograph,[7] and organized and chaired their study sections (both in the United States and the United Kingdom).

No doubt, I have benefited from these professional societies and institutions. Though I faced many obstacles, and though my research often swam against the current, I also had what some have described as the most prestigious position in the country in professional nutritional science. I was a tenured full professor holding an endowed chair in the top-ranked nutritional

---

* I was invited by the ACS vice president at that time, John Stevens, to the panel chaired by Alan Vegotsky. Unfortunately, I had to quit after a couple of years because I had become overwhelmed by other projects. Both Stevens and Vegotsky were generous to invite me.

† Other support came from (1) the Chinese Academies of Preventive Medicine and Medical Sciences under the direction of Drs. Chen Junshi and Li Junyao, respectively—who provided approximately 300 person-years of professional labor, including twenty person-years from senior Chinese scientists (funded by the World Bank) to work in my laboratory at Cornell; (2) twenty-four research laboratories in six countries that analyzed biological samples; and (3) the Clinical Trials Unit of the Radcliffe Infirmary of Oxford University under the direction of Sir Richard Peto and Dr. Jill Boreham.

science department in the United States, where I conducted the largest, best-funded, most-published project in the department.* And so I do not question the legitimacy of these institutions lightly, or as one embittered by a lifetime of exclusion. I am concerned for the public and for the integrity of these institutions, if such a thing has ever existed, precisely because I have been up close and personal enough to see where that integrity should have resulted in an intervention, but did not.

The sense that our institutions are not living up to their potential is a common concern today, and public trust in our institutions seems to be at an all-time low. This is especially clear in the public's attitudes toward higher education, the media, government, and science itself. Sadly, this may be the new norm. Opinions that once would have been dismissed as unbelievably jaded or paranoid are now commonplace. With that environment in mind, I worry that many readers will wade through the examples of this section with a greater feeling of numbness than of anger. I worry that we have become far too desensitized to manipulation, censorship, and dishonesty—that few are surprised to hear that corporate interests underwrite our collective understanding of nutrition—and that what I've written here is hardly an anomaly.

Nevertheless, judging by comments I've heard, and the way media report on this issue (or fail to report), very few know the tremendous extent of industry influences—from self-serving research funding and financially rewarding consultancies, to the conniving ruthlessness with which these influences operate beyond public awareness. This is why I've focused on various examples from my own career throughout this book. Although some of them have been mentioned in previous books, and although I sometimes feel uncomfortable discussing them, I feel very strongly that they are instructive in this new context. I've had the strange fortune of being able to "live in the dirt"—to work very closely with these institutions. The public deserves to know how their tax dollars are being spent, how their health is being affected, and how dominant perspectives are being shaped, be it in Washington, DC, or in the classrooms of "higher" education. Moreover, even if this kind of industry influence has become normalized to the point of our

---

* According to the director of the financial office of Cornell's Division of Nutritional Sciences.

numbness, that doesn't make it any more acceptable. The things we know about nutrition and health should be determined by evidence alone, not by the spending power of food and drug industries.

I'm tired of living in the dirt.

#2: PROTECT AND RESTORE ACADEMIC FREEDOM

This second recommendation for how to improve our institutions goes hand in hand with the first. For my part, without academic freedom, my career would have starved in the ditch decades ago. I never would have written *Whole*, or *The China Study* before it. I certainly wouldn't be writing this book now, inviting you to question the role of institutions.

Academic freedom has been an important part of intellectual life for centuries, and tenure has long been the tool used to protect this freedom. The modern system of academic tenure in the United States, which grants qualified professors the right to hold a position indefinitely, was conceived in 1915, established in 1940 as a Statement of Principles on Academic Freedom and Tenure,[8] and updated in 1970. Similar to Supreme Court justices, the lifelong appointments protected by tenure are meant to safeguard professors' freedom of speech and investigation, no matter what pressure internal or external interests might exert on the university. Of course, tenure hasn't always worked as perfectly as it should. As with anything, the ideals at which it aims are not always perfectly implemented. Some detractors of tenure argue that it encourages complacency and laziness among protected professors. But I think these risks are often overstated, particularly when compared to the alternative. Without the protection of tenure, academic freedom is far too vulnerable to manipulation and corruption.

Moreover, tenured positions are not granted lightly. Tenure is generally granted after an assistant professor is promoted to associate professor after seven years of observation, and includes an intensive review by a committee of peers. Thereafter, an associate professor may be further promoted to full professor after another seven to fifteen years. Clearly tenure is not won quickly or easily. It requires ambition. So long as the university is rigorous in these procedures, the kind of people who earn tenured professorships are unlikely to be lazy or complacent, as the critique often goes.

I earned tenure when I was on the faculty of Virginia Tech at the age of thirty-five. Fortunately, my tenure was reconfirmed six years later when I took a position at Cornell. Of all the professional events throughout my career, this relatively early achievement of tenure was surely one of the most important. It prevented numerous efforts to silence me or get me fired. Just to give one example, a request for my termination was once sent by the chairman of the Egg Board (a national poultry-industry advocacy group) to the Cornell University president, Dale Corson, and the dean of the College of Agriculture, David Call. These men knew me well—in fact, Corson had interviewed me, along with Dean Call's predecessor, Keith Kennedy, when I was first recruited to my position at Cornell in 1974—but even if they had not, tenure would have ensured my protection.

Of course, tenure cannot protect the deviant academic from *all* forms of outside threat, or from ridicule and contempt. As crucial as job security and academic freedom is, it cannot guard absolutely against all forms of personal attacks. But despite its shortcomings, it has still played an important role in protecting academic freedom. In my case, even when the directors of Cornell's Division of Nutrition Sciences were disgruntled by the work I was doing, my job remained secure. Even when private interests demanded that I be fired, my publicly funded research thrived.

What's become of these safeguards? They are declining. The following chart shows that among basic science departments in US medical schools, in a span of only nineteen years (1980–1999), the number of tenure-based faculty positions dropped 33 percent. As of 2004, tenure-track positions were outnumbered by non–tenure track positions.[9] In the time since, tenure has disintegrated even further. Is it any surprise that academic freedom has been neutered, and the search for truth censored and policed?

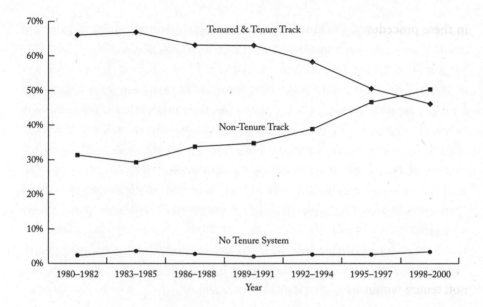

The decrease in tenure isn't the only threat to academic freedom. On April 30, 2018, the Associated Press published a news item titled "Documents Show Ties Between University, Conservative Donors," which exposes the ways in which big money donors have compromised universities' public responsibility to objectively search for the truth.[10] The article begins:

> *Virginia's largest public university granted the conservative Charles Koch Foundation a say in the hiring and firing of professors in exchange for millions of dollars in donations, according to newly released documents. The release of donor agreements between George Mason University and the foundation follows years of denials by university administrators that the Koch donations inhibit academic freedom.*

This information was only publicized after a judge's order commanded its disclosure, which the university opposed for years. It details how the Koch Foundation exerted considerable influence on campus through their right to name two of five members on a faculty hiring committee. Further, the Koch Foundation "enjoyed similar appointment rights to advisory panels that had the right . . . to recommend firing a professor who failed to live up to standards." But fear not! The university assures the public and its students that such donations did not "inhibit academic freedom." Don't you trust them?

A few days later, the *New York Times* told much the same story, elaborating on a surprising breadth of corporate interests infiltrating academic spaces across the country.[11] To be fair, both the university and the Koch Foundation would likely point out that these agreements have since expired. Nevertheless, given that not every existing agreement is available for public scrutiny, and that this one was deliberately hidden from the public for years, it's very difficult to believe that similarly cozy relationships don't persist in some form or another.

Some may argue that this donor–institution relationship is simply "business as usual" and therefore nothing to be concerned about. I would grant this point halfway: such relationships certainly do reflect a businesslike, transactional arrangement. However, they need not and should not be the norm. Others may also defend donors' right to influence how their money is spent, especially when their influence is limited to minority memberships on such committees. But after numerous experiences and decades in academia, I know that minority membership on such "academic" committees doesn't have a minority impact. It is almost impossible to quantify and control conflicts of interest in this way. Even if the institution is represented on such advisory committees with a majority of members, the mere presence of those donor-appointees and the implicit knowledge that future funding may be in the balance puts the university's representatives in an impossible situation. More often than not, they will feel a strong pressure to serve the donors' interests, even if it goes against the university's mission to serve the public.

Claims of impartiality and academic integrity should also be questioned in individual research projects. Is it even possible for researchers and their administrators to uphold their institution's claim of credibility and objectivity when participating in a blatantly industry-funded research project? Let's face it, this system serves donors like the Koch Foundation extremely well. So long as academic institutions are willing to pimp the credibility of their hallowed names (for approximately $50 million, in the case of George Mason), certain research interests will be satisfied, and certain researchers will be hired, while the rest are left behind.

This is not a convoluted conspiracy, but rather a case of very simple economics. Such dealings seriously contradict universities' claims that they are the seekers of truth and the protectors of intellectual freedom. Worst of all is the impact this industry entanglement has on the public, whose own tax contributions do not confer influence of equal proportion. I'm reminded here of how the Communications Office at Cornell was blocked from publicizing the success of our online plant-based nutrition certificate course, which is based on decades' worth of *taxpayer-funded* research. The university was happy enough to let the course partner with its online program, eCornell, but not to publicize its successes, for . . . what? Fear of losing donor funding from impacted industries?

We need to ask ourselves, as a society, whether our academies' credibility should be bought and sold; whether a donation to a public institution should be conditional on private interests and for how long; and whether academic freedom, public trust, and even freedom of speech can and should be transformed into mere bargaining chips.

I wish these comments were unnecessary. Many will say they're obvious. And yet I worry for the next generation of scientists interested in conducting research that cuts against the grain of orthodoxy, such as the unusually far-reaching and fundamental effects of animal protein consumption on disease outcomes like cancer and heart disease. I worry they won't be allowed to ask such questions in the first place—that today's setting is even less conducive to that kind of research than it was in my time. If we fail to protect and restore academic freedom, how will we ever protect and preserve the interchange of useful, controversial research subjects?

#3: RESCUE SCIENCE FROM TECHNOLOGY AND INDUSTRY

Many would agree that the purpose of science is different from the purpose of technology. But what are those purposes, and why is the distinction important? Science, in my view, is the art of observation, and its purpose is the pursuit of knowledge, which has no hard borders or obvious endpoints. It pursues that realm of knowledge beyond our consciousness. Technology, on the other hand, is a constructive venture concerned with the creation of products that solve problems. Ideally, scientists pursue what they do not yet know. They often embark on the scientific journey without even knowing all of the questions worth asking. After all, if they already knew, the exercise would be pointless. Technologists, on the other hand, generally pursue solutions to identifiable problems. They are not led by the unknown, but by questions they have already determined to be important. How can we make this system function more efficiently? How can we solve this problem, plug that gap, transform this task? Oftentimes, science precedes technology, though of course technology can also aid in the scientific process.

The reason I make this distinction between science and technology is because I have seen many fields of science transformed to instead resemble technology over the course of my career, including nutrition. "Scientists" in the field of nutrition have become less and less interested in the unknown and in questions they haven't yet considered. The kinds of questions most acceptable in nutrition "science" today are those with predetermined importance: How can we get enough protein? How can we create and use a more perfect index to quantify and catalog nutrient density? How can we lower serum cholesterol levels? Perhaps these questions do not sound so bad, but serious problems arise when they are the only questions being asked and virtually no one questions their fundamental usefulness. A clear, specific example of technology's grip on nutrition is the reductionist research on nutrients out of context, based on the belief that out-of-context nutrients can be produced (as supplements) in order to solve problems (nutrient deficiencies) and make money as a bonus.

In short, nutrition science has yielded to the purposes of technology. It has shed its open-minded, interrogative character in favor of analytic problem-solving, wherein the problems have (mostly) already been determined and the tools for solving them are limited. In many ways, contemporary nutrition has become the *antithesis* of science. It is not alone in this regard—many fields of science have succumbed to technology to a certain extent—but being part of a larger group does not make the change in the field any less significant or concerning.

WFPB nutrition doesn't jibe well with the nutrition "science" of the establishment. It doesn't jibe well precisely because it is no technology at all. Whole foods are not produced in the same sense that pills are produced.

Whole foods are not technological solutions (unless you imagine a technologist creator). Moreover, even the conditions for *creating* whole foods (fertile earth, rain, sunshine, etc.) do not require production. These conditions and "products" already exist. They have been determined and fine-tuned—whether by miraculous Nature or by some combination of cosmic coincidence and inexplicable luck—and these already-existing conditions do not demand the influence of technologists. This isn't to say that technology hasn't exerted its influence over the food system. Agricultural practice today is nothing if not technological practice; farmers today have had to become technologists, their earnings entirely dependent on heavy machinery and the "get big or get out" logic of our technologist utopia. But WFPB nutrition itself is *not* a technological solution—quite the opposite, in fact—and so it generates little interest or funding support from the techno-scientific establishment.

I don't pretend to be a scholar on the philosophy of science, only a long-time researcher who greatly enjoyed his career in science. Science as I knew it offered me an extraordinary opportunity to be my own boss, to explore a wide and fascinating range of research questions, and to follow them wherever they might lead. I was held accountable by my professional peers, who judged my applications for funding and manuscripts for publication. Naturally, they were often skeptical, and this led to much civil debate, as science should. Without this skepticism and debate my scientific career would have been far less meaningful and productive. But this kind of open and civil debate has, increasingly, gone missing from the field of nutrition.

Unlike technology, research is not and should not be a product, but a work in progress. It is a process by which we negotiate a more accurate and useful view of the world: posing, reframing, and discovering new questions along the way. Some researchers prefer to work on very specific findings in depth, perhaps for many years, until their quantitative characteristics and validity are firmly established; others prefer experiments that simultaneously examine breadth, depth, and context of effect. In either case, hypotheses are being tested throughout, until time or funding runs out. Seldom can we rest our views on the results of a single experiment, and never do we run out of questions worth asking.

In the world of technology, a product either succeeds or fails in doing what it sets out to do. This success or failure is relatively easy to test and improve upon. *Not so in science.* In science we thrust ourselves open-minded into the observable unknown, and we must be careful when we do so. If we begin our research with preconceived ideas about failure or success, then we have already lost our way, for failure and success are value judgments altogether separate from the act of observation. In technology, there tends to be a clear horizon toward which our work is aimed, whereas in science, the horizon is vague and distant. I don't mean to suggest that science should not be interpreted and put to good use; eventually we should look back on what we have observed and make decisions about relevant behavior and future questions. But to muddle our observation with value judgments *about* the observation is to slip into the role of one who is seeking a specific outcome, and this is not science.

Make no mistake, technology can enrich our lives. The very book in your hands (or on your screen, or in your ears) is an example of technology; books are a solution to the puzzle of how to transmit language across space and time, and obviously have had a tremendous impact on the development of our species. Likewise, technology has a role in promoting health and wellness. If I were to fracture my femur and end up in the hospital, I certainly wouldn't protest against the X-ray machine. But when it comes to nutrition and diseases that are regulated by nutrition, I believe we must be able to look beyond technology, and fund accordingly.

This requires a significant shift in thought. If the modern prominence of the word *nutraceutical* (describing a food or food product that assists in preventing or treating disease) tells us anything, it is that we are not currently disentangling nutrition and technology, but rather entangling them further. *Nutraceutical* is, on a linguistic level, a celebration of nutrients as drugs—in other words, nutrition-as-technology. Indeed, I fear that the word is often used to lend greater emphasis to nutrition as a serious "science." By importing the connotations attached to the miraculous technology of pharmaceutical medicine, nutrition is supposed to seem more potent and important. But nutrients are *not* drugs, and the concept of *nutraceutical* is a whole lot of nothing—a cloud of smoke, a bridge to nowhere.

Although the science of wholistic nutrition may comfortably coexist alongside the technology of X-ray machines, wholistic nutrition is incompatible with our notion of nutrition-as-technology.

SCIENCE IN CORPORATE CLOTHES

As a result of this blurred line between science and technology, science has also become increasingly entangled with industry, which demands technology as a means to profit. We need look no further than the development of dietary guidelines in the United States to see how this industry-technology-science entanglement plays out. Since 1980, the US Department of Agriculture (USDA) and the US Department of Health and Human Services (HHS) have jointly sponsored the development of these guidelines. The USDA is undeniably influenced by the livestock industry. Indeed, its primary purpose has always been to serve American agriculture, ever since its establishment in 1862. This isn't a bad thing, on its face (the interests of American farmers *should* be represented and valued), but things have changed tremendously since 1862. American agriculture today is not the small family farm of old that remains in my soul; instead, it is huge agribusinesses geared toward maximally efficient production of livestock and related crops, all for the sake of achieving maximum profit, not maximum health. (Just as the science of nutrition has become increasingly focused on technology, so has agriculture.) And so, when the USDA sets out to make dietary guidelines, how could we expect to see recommendations that might undermine the technology of American agribusiness, regardless of what the science says? As long as the governing body is entangled with industry, so will its recommendations be entangled with industry interests. Meanwhile, HHS, the other partner in the development of US Dietary Guidelines, is similarly influenced by the pharmaceutical industry. This should come as no surprise—how could the HHS not be influenced by the pharmaceutical industry when our entire concept of *health* and our system of maintaining it is centered on the use of pills and procedures?

Perhaps to give the impression of fairness and transparency, the Dietary Guidelines Advisory Committee gives the public a modest opportunity to comment on the updated guidelines, released every five years by a science advisory committee. For the most recent report, the public had seventy-five days to comment.[12] Many people are impressed when they hear about this process. I'm not one of them. Appearances of public participation aside, the entire system is politically controlled. First, members chosen for the science advisory committee tend to be disinclined to challenge corporate interests.

Indeed, they often have industry-based personal conflicts of interest. Second, the final report made available for public comment must be approved by the secretary of agriculture, who is neither an expert on the science nor a likely candidate to keep a watchful eye on the livestock industry, to which they are indebted and to which they must ultimately report.

I have closely followed the evolution of this program ever since my friends and colleagues Professor Mark Hegsted of Harvard and Allan Forbes at the FDA wrote the first Dietary Guidelines report in 1980 in an office next to mine. Likewise, I have served on several similar policy panels. Thus, in May 2015, when the seventy-five-day public comment period was open for comment, I submitted a properly referenced 773-word commentary,[13] with thirty-three professional references, making several points that I believed had been overlooked in the proposed 2015–2020 report. Among the 29,000 comments the report received, the well-recognized Congressional newspaper *The Hill* (distributed throughout Congressional offices) highlighted my remarks on their front page. I was temporarily encouraged that my commentary was receiving so much attention, but the USDA group ignored it.*

In the "Strategies for Action" listed in the most recent guidelines (2015–2020),[12] the authors encourage the "[promotion,] development and availability of food products that align with the *Dietary Guidelines* in food retail and food service establishments." The intent of this particular guideline assumes that (1) the USDA guidelines are in a position to encourage "beneficial" change, (2) industry will yield to their efforts, and most importantly, (3) their influence is being exerted unidirectionally, *from* the guidelines and *toward* industry. I take a different view of the matter. Clearly, given the practices of the past twenty to thirty years, the guidelines yield to the influence of industry just as much, if not far more, than industry yields to the guidelines.

In case you think I'm being naïve or unrealistic to expect sound dietary guidelines free of industry influence, consider this: Canada limited industry

---

* Among other recommendations, I suggested that (1) they cite Esselstyn's and Ornish's heart disease reversal evidence, since the report implied there was no such research; (2) they comment on the effect of nutrition on cancer (their comments were virtually nil); and (3) they note that the cost of health care, as currently practiced in the US, is the highest in the world but the health return on that investment is the lowest.

input when developing its 2019 Food Guide[14] and it resulted in a refreshing step in the right direction of favoring the public. Recommendations include "choose protein foods that come from plants more often . . . you don't need to eat large amounts of protein foods to meet your nutritional needs . . . [and] make water your drink of choice." Other changes, quite remarkably, include doing away with

> *recommendations for specific portions or daily servings . . . "Nobody really followed [these], nobody knew what a serving size was . . ." said [Dr. Yoni] Freedhof . . . "But they provided the food industry with something really powerful to market—especially the dairy industry, which talked about how many servings of dairy you needed to have per day, and how Canadians were doing a poor job with that."*

In my view, Canada's recommendations don't go far enough to promote the *optimum* diet; there are parts worthy of critique, based on the science. But they deserve great credit for their attempts to reduce industry influence over this process. Among those complaining about the publication are the Dairy Farmers of Canada[14]—a good sign, I think. Maybe someday if the US Dietary Guidelines can extricate themselves from the grip of industry, we may read about similar dissent from the National Livestock Producers Association and other special interest groups that prey on the health of Americans.

* * *

When we strip away the purposes of technology and the influence of industry, what are we left with? What is science capable of, when freed from these twin anchors? It depends. I'm not going to categorically defend *all* science for the sake of science. The value of scientific hypotheses, which might eventually become scientific theories, depends on a number of things. Even the most intelligent study design and most precise measurements, for example, do not guarantee great relevancy. Nevertheless, given the right conditions, science is capable of achieving much more than science-as-technology and science-as-industry.

If we are a society that cares about our members' well-being and our future, we must decide whether we value the unobstructed freedom of science, and whether we believe in its integrity. Far too much of today's "science" is bound to external factors. Practical decisions on policy, regulations, and marketing are made on the basis of protecting business, promoting the status quo, patronizing the public, paying the bills, and keeping the peace. Even when science is produced independently, not beholden to outside interests, and funded entirely by the public, it may struggle for recognition. This completely undermines its value. For although science as an art of observation can be fascinating in its own right, its true usefulness comes later, when competing interpretations are brought forward for cross examination and we glean insight for making life decisions. Debate, conducted with civility, is paramount.

So long as science is caught in the grips of technology and industry, however, that considerate debate will not receive the attention it deserves, and our "science" will continue to fall short of its potential.

#4: HEAL NUTRITION

In addition to the three more general recommendations above, which could apply to more than one field of science, or even to life beyond science, I offer these more specific recommendations for the field of nutrition. They comprise a culmination of all the issues I've discussed—a healing protocol, meant to be informed by science-as-science:

1. Construct an efficacious nutritional science education program for all accredited medical school curricula. Medical institutions that fail to offer adequate training in nutrition science should not receive government support. Adequate training is best obtained both by classroom instruction and by a practicum (perhaps using the WFPB diet for a period of at least two weeks and monitoring results in an abbreviated lab assessment).
2. Develop reimbursement procedures for primary care physicians who apply this education in nutrition. This current omission is a personal, professional, institutional, societal, and moral disgrace.

3. Establish a new National Institute for Nutrition (to join the current twenty-seven NIH institutes).
4. Transform food subsidy programs to encourage food production that aligns with reliable nutritional evidence and consumer protection.
5. Create a food and nutrition advisory council that truly serves the interests of the consumer and that is financed by an endowment trust fund beyond the influence of corporate financial interests.

Here we must be brave. Returning to the idea of science-as-science, in the field of nutrition, will result in a great deal of disruption. But then, this disruption is exactly the point. Ironically, one of the closest parallels to this kind of disruption comes from the world of technology. "Disruptive technology" is an emerging technology that significantly alters the way business is conducted, even to the point of rendering old technologies obsolete. An example of a potentially useful disruptive technology in medicine is artificial intelligence (AI). According to a research group from Stanford, "Recent advancements in deep learning and large datasets have enabled algorithms to surpass the performance of medical professionals in a wide variety of medical imaging tasks, including diabetic retinopathy detection,[15] skin cancer classification,[16] and arrhythmia detection."[17] Thus, in the case of AI in medicine, disruptive technology threatens to replace human experts in the task of diagnosing disease, offering in exchange more technically accurate diagnoses.

But WFPB nutrition does not deserve the label "disruptive technology," for it is no technology at all, and so here I twist the phrase. A more apt title for WFPB nutrition is *disruptive science*. WFPB nutrition threatens to disrupt many industries—pharmaceutical, food production, clinical care, hospitalization—and these industries are well aware of this threat. If WFPB nutrition were adopted on a wide scale, many jobs in these industries would be lost and many fortunes would be threatened. But we should not let that uncomfortable fact impede improvements to our health. Or are we so unsure of our ability to innovate in new directions?

I for one would like to cast my ballot for disruption. I know of no positive change that did not disrupt what came before it. And surely nutritional ignorance, which has done so much damage and so thoroughly pervades the entire biomedical research and clinical practice system, deserves disruption. Malnutrition is unquestionably the number one cause of death, the number one cause of high runaway costs, and more recently, the number one cause of environmental catastrophe. If we ignore this last consequence, everything else that I've written here will be wasted breath. Therefore, in the spirit of survival, I reiterate this final recommendation for the future: heal nutrition.

COULD CHANGING OUR DIETS DEFEAT COVID-19?

This book was mostly complete by early 2020, except for editing, which took place until late July. During that time, the novel coronavirus crisis arrived, followed by an unprecedented disruption of our lives. Jobs have been lost, educational institutions from pre-K to universities have been closed, events attracting crowds have been canceled and prohibited, and businesses have been shuttered around the world. I feel my work here would be incomplete if I did not take a moment to ask whether this book's central message applies to viral diseases like COVID-19.

Briefly, it does! And I believe it has the power to make a huge difference in both this crisis and future viral epidemics and pandemics. Although elementary yet practical actions like wearing face masks, washing our hands frequently, disinfecting public surfaces, and maintaining social distancing in public places are understandable and necessary, I believe there is a much more empowering and untold story here about the power of nutrition. If we don't pay closer attention to that story—and soon!—I fear that we risk our existence on this planet.

There are many obstacles in conveying this information to our families, friends, and the public. The combined size of the agriculture, food, drug, and medical infrastructure industries make up a huge proportion of our total economy, and it is not in their best interests to encourage sweeping dietary change. I have seen their power in action many times throughout my career, as described throughout this book. My view on this power dynamic is the same as it ever has been—I have no interest in proactively coercing others to listen to my advice, or the industry-sanctioned "guidance" of seemingly authoritative institutions, because I am reasonably convinced that people can and should make their own choices. There are certainly other obstacles that need to be addressed, including racial and economic disparities in medical care and food access, but the larger point remains: we have to give the public *all* the credible information on nutrition and disease, including that which threatens industry, much of which I know after being in this business for sixty-five years.

The information I have in mind related to the coronavirus pandemic is professionally obtained, peer-reviewed published data from a study in rural China that I organized in the early 1980s and directed with some exceptional colleagues from China and the University of Oxford. It was conducted in 1983[1] (involving 130 villages and 6,500 adults 35–64 years of age) and repeated in 1989[2] (when 16 areas in Taiwan were added to 138 villages in China, totaling 8,900 individuals). An unparalleled quantity of data was collected on disease mortality rates, lifestyle, diet, and nutrition (by recording food intake and taking blood serum samples). I've already discussed some of this information in my previous books, but the most interesting data given the current crisis involve four viruses and their relationships to various cancers. In particular, we studied hepatitis B (HBV), a primary cause of liver cancer, in particular depth.

Before going further, I must address a fundamental but often misunderstood idea about viruses: that they are all vastly different. On the one hand, they are different, and each virus strain creates its own unique symptoms. But also, critically, all share something in common. The process by which viruses invade us, and the process by which our immune system works to create a defense, custom-making antibodies and related actors for each virus strain are, by and large, the same across viruses.

With that in mind, four sets of statistically significant correlations were obtained on this HBV virus. There were two datasets on the associations of plant food factors with the prevalence of antibodies and antigens, and two on the associations of markers of animal food consumption on the prevalence of these same antibodies and antigens.[2]

Each dataset consistently and independently supported the same conclusion: plant-based food consumption was associated with more antibodies and fewer antigens, while markers of animal-based food consumption were associated with the opposite—fewer antibodies and more antigens. Quite remarkably, even small amounts of animal-based foods (compared to the average amounts consumed in the US) produced this effect and, further, these small amounts were also highly correlated with liver cancer death rates ($P < 0.001$). Vegetable consumption, specifically, was highly correlated with higher prevalence of antibodies ($P < 0.001$). In other words, plant-based food favored immunity. Conversely, animal-based food favored death.

Our laboratory animal studies added further support for the association of animal-food consumption with liver cancer mortality. Mice, genetically programmed to develop liver cancer begun by the HBV virus, did so only when animal protein was increased above the minimum amount of protein needed for good health. The results were striking and were observed both histologically and biochemically.[3-5]

I suggest with considerable confidence that these findings apply to COVID-19 as well, especially for older individuals whose health is already compromised by diseases related to nutrition, such as heart disease and other chronic degenerative diseases, a well-known effect that is called co-morbidity. Using a whole food, plant-based diet throughout one's life should lessen the susceptibility to COVID-19 while simultaneously increasing COVID-19 antibodies, a win-win effect. Based on other studies, this latter immune response may begin within days, possibly providing enough time for people not yet infected by COVID-19 to strengthen their immunity.

Furthermore, this dietary practice should be maintained because there are recent but unsubstantiated news reports that some people who have been infected may become reinfected. If this is confirmed, then dietary lifestyle changes would represent not only a way of being prepared but also of *staying* prepared.

To conclude, then, even though there is no direct proof of a COVID-19–nutrition link, I am quite confident *that this nutritional strategy could produce a faster, safer, and more comprehensive long-term program for coping with viral diseases like COVID-19,* for it bolsters overall immunity and many of the viral-specific processes just discussed. If I am correct in this, then I submit that in the future, as soon as we learn the genetic identity of new viruses and develop effective testing procedures, we will not need to impose social practices beyond those customarily used for transmissible illnesses. Neither will we feel so helpless as we await the development of extraordinarily expensive drugs and vaccines with variable levels of efficacy and safety.

Incidentally, even just since I began writing this postscript, David Gelles and Jesse Drucker have published a relevant article in the *New York Times* about the corporate race for a coronavirus vaccine.[6] Billions of dollars—some from private venture capital, but much of it provided by the taxpayer—now flow like water, with great hopes of developing a vaccine. Even organizations that have never developed a drug before are jumping on board, as hype and false claims continue to mount. These efforts are predicated, above all else, on what the article rightly calls a "desperate public." Consistently missing from this and similar commentaries is the suggestion that individuals of the public might control their own destinies.

To summarize, I draw my confidence in this suggestion both from the empirical evidence cited here and from an abundance of evidence showing the comprehensive effect of whole food, plant-based nutrition on total health. As always, I would emphasize that the nutritional effect I propose here is that obtained from whole foods, not from isolated nutrients contained therein.

And finally, I see this frightening experience with COVID-19 as an opportunity to implement the grander message on nutrition and the role that it plays throughout our society. The time to take advantage of this opportunity, as costly as it has been, is NOW. Let's get something in return for that cost!

AFTERWORD

NATURE GETS THE LAST WORD

Often, nonfiction books conclude with a call to action (CTA). This is where the author prescribes a next step to the reader. The quality of a CTA can be quantified by calculating the conversion rate: the percentage of readers who take the desired action. Information about nutrition may be followed by all sorts of CTAs: Register for our conference! Purchase our plan! Buy our miraculous multivitamin that captures all the wonderful health properties of the Amazon rainforest! These repulsive examples illustrate how thin the veil has become between everyday communication and the logic of marketing. In our society, it seems we cannot even conclude a narrative about health and personal well-being without relying on marketing gimmicks.

When it comes to health and nutrition, I've grown weary of the simplistic CTA format. Given the complexity and perplexity that pervade these subjects, CTAs are insufficient, and they remind me of regimentation, of goose-step behavior. I fear that there's too much action, too much knee-jerk reaction, too many advertisements and con men trying to sell another product. There is a blizzard of confusing diet and nutritional information, even backed by "evidence," all of which the public is asked to act on. Hypothetically, one could even find "evidence" for the disaster that is the standard American diet (or, ironically, SAD). The missing key is discernment. Amid all these calls to action, neither the producers of evidence (professionals in nutrition and medicine) nor their dependents (the public) attend to the *quality* of evidence that action is based on. Neither are they equipped to translate the foreign language of science—much like single-minded scientists working in their respective silos.

If I might offer an alternative, it is this: a call to greater care and deliberation in our actions. I am not suggesting there should be no action, either collective or individual, for those who wish to challenge the diseased status quo and transform our society's troubled relationship with health. There are organizations doing such work that I am proud to endorse, and from which I receive no compensation, listed at the end of this commentary.

But in the meantime, moving forward, I'd like to suggest the following:

A call to critical reflection. Reflection on our past, the institutional limits that bind us, the myths that impact our perspective on health, and the way we define science itself. Reflection on how institutions came to dominate the many fields of disease research and treatment, and reflection on the severe consequences of that dominance. For well over a hundred years, we have been sold costly, toxic pharmaceutical responses to disease. To reiterate just a couple of examples mentioned earlier: the majority of authorized cancer drugs (57 percent) between 2009 and 2013 came to market *without any evidence* that "they improved the quality or quantity of patients' lives,"[1] and five-year survival rates for patients using cytotoxic chemotherapy drugs increased by an average of only 2.1 percent,[2] a significant portion of which may simply be placebo. This ineffectiveness is nothing new. Recall from the history that there was no promising evidence when these "solutions" were first devised. Reflect on why we went forward with those protocols anyway. How did we come to regard poison as a tool in the pursuit of health? Ineptitude and ignorance may play a part, but so does arrogance. Remember that old surgeon's critique, that only the timid "who fear the knife" could possibly object to surgery. Remember also those whose power and wealth depend on the knife.

Reflect on where we are, individually and collectively, in the greater timeline of our evolution. Reflect on how stagnant we have been in certain areas. Why do we continue to celebrate "high-quality" animal protein, when so much evidence suggests that the foods containing it are killing us? When experimental laboratory animal studies, human intervention trials, and international correlation studies all suggest the same conclusion, why do we continue to celebrate that myth? Why do we continue to focus on individual nutrients, as in nutrient density and nutrient supplements? Why do we count calories to control body weight, but ignore the broader effects of food? And reflect on how we are impacting the environment. Scientists tell us that we are in the midst of the sixth mass extinction—not in the near future, but now. Will we be complacent and quicken it, or will we reflect on how our behavior is fueling it? Are we capable of this kind of honesty? We are being spoon-fed the apocalypse, but for what purpose and by whose directive? Is it really worth preserving an insatiable hunger for profit and for foods that have devastating effects on personal and planetary health? Do we really value the almighty market more than survival? Do we prefer market-enforced overconsumption, or would we rather consume sustainably? If we do not reflect on these threats, then Nature will get the last word. There will be no more calls to action delivered in the way we have grown accustomed to. Nature, which is far more resilient than any one species, may continue to issue its own calls, but our species will not be around to hear them.

A call to authentic conversation—about the scientific evidence; about the things we value, such as academic freedom and transparent policy development; about the future we're headed toward. Conversation for the betterment of our communities. These are not solely academic debates. If we can only ever think of them as academic debates of little practical relevance, then our society will never improve its relationship with health, education, and power. We should not foist all responsibility for our actions, for our health, on professional "experts." Too often, they are virtually unschooled in the science of nutrition, are susceptible to corruption and manipulation, and do not communicate well with the public. If all hope of progress is left stranded in their academic halls and policy boardrooms, then that hope is nothing more than a pipe dream.

There is far more hope in the behavior of everyday people, but only if we take our behavior to the visible spaces of our society. Let local businesses know that there is a demand for nutritious options, and raise hell about the vampiric corporations that manufacture addictive foods that leave us malnourished. There are both loud and quiet ways to raise hell. If picketing before the plastic battlements of Wendy's[3] isn't for you, then at least protest their power over your bank account. Even simpler, always align your life's practices with the message you wish to communicate. If health is truly important to you, then be diligent in how you pursue that health. If the health of our society and planet are important to you, great! But do not let those seemingly insurmountable goals distract you from the aspect of health most in your control. Remember your own agency. Begin with your own family, your own health. As much as our society extols the importance of finding good role models, the inward-facing labor of *becoming* a good role model—a potent form of activism—is too often overlooked.

A call to authentic conversation is a call to healthy social function. The more isolated and antisocial we are, the more fractured our discourse is, and the more fractured our discourse, the more damaging it becomes. Industry is always trying to sell the narrative of isolation. Their advertisements target our greatest social and psychological insecurities. They tell us that we are alone, unloved, incomplete. That we are lonely individuals in need of a fix that only they can give us. This narrative perpetuates their power, but it is a mirage. We are *not* isolated. Authentic conversation about health and nutrition, and about our values more broadly, both within and beyond our communities, is the best way to prove that fact.

A call to civil disagreement. Communicate civilly—that is, in an open and respectful way. Address the science as honestly and candidly as possible; address dishonesty in the same way. Let the spirit of science, of skepticism, guide your judgment, but do not use it as an excuse to never engage in the first place. In that spirit, I will gladly consider any alternate interpretation to the evidence presented in this book. No, more than consider it—I invite it. I would find it very disheartening if mine were the last words on this issue, for "last words" have no place in science. Even as I conducted my research, I often wrestled with skepticism. *Can it really be that this information is real, that the miraculous health properties claimed for animal foods, foods that are a part of my personal and cultural heritage, have been overstated or, even worse, that these foods can cause cancer and other metabolic diseases?* Knitting together the many provocative findings of my research, and the findings of others, eventually led me to a fundamentally different perspective on how nutrition is defined. But this perspective deserves and requires further consideration. To the skeptics, I say come forth, and if you have something to say, let us hear it. Your silence is no great benefit to me or to society.

Disagree civilly with other members of the public, too. Meet with people where they are (it's the only place we *can* meet them!) and discuss the profound effects of nutrition on health. Over the past two decades, I have been blown away by the number of people who have approached me in public to say that they gave the WFPB diet a try and saw profound effects. These are not stories that we should hide from each other, or avoid simply because diet is a sensitive topic. Be respectful, of course, but if you are one of the many people who have gotten off of numerous medications and shocked your doctor by merely changing the foods you put into your body, then the world can only benefit from hearing your story. I would even say that the empowered have a responsibility to share their power, whether by example or by thoughtful engagement.

A call to recognition and acceptance. Acceptance of Nature and acceptance of ourselves (as if there's any division between the two!). Recognition of the guiding principles of Nature, whose essence is wholism. Recall the experimental research results introduced in chapter eight, which so profoundly affected my journey in science. For more than a decade, our research focused on trying to find the *one* biological mechanism for the promotion of cancer growth by animal protein. Lo and behold, there was no single mechanism, but rather many, all working in a highly integrated way on different parts of this complex process, *but all to the same end*. Animal protein increased the activities of mechanisms that favor cancer growth and decreased mechanisms that prevent cancer growth. This integration, when considered in the context of the body's ever-changing mechanistic activities, explains both the promotion of cancer by animal protein and a more general means by which nutrients cause wholistic biological effects. This nutritional effect demonstrates the ineffectiveness of reductionist, drug-dependent control of health. Perhaps most miraculously, this wholistic wisdom is the body's *default*. Instant by instant, the body restores and maintains homeostasis, the technical term for biological harmony.

I see no reason why wholism's guiding principles—appreciation for context, communication, integration—should not be scaled up to change our world. Why should they not someday serve as the basis for all interpersonal relations? Why should they not influence social organization at all levels? Just as colonies of cells with a common purpose within organs perform specific tasks as parts of a greater whole, and just as organs with a common purpose coordinate their work within the context of a greater whole, groups of people ought to be able to work together with a common purpose in a way that honors the whole. By sharing talents, communicating openly, and honoring the greater context from which we come, we can improve the health of our communities and protect the health of the planet. There are many platforms freely available today to easily establish local groups and organizations. Social media, though riddled with many problems, can be a powerful tool in this regard. If we use it wisely, and alongside more traditional methods of organization, to discuss collective action within our communities, then such action may follow. If we instead imagine that these problems are insurmountable, distant, and abstract, then they will remain just that. What is there to stop one concerned parent from joining another, to discuss the damaging effects of the USDA's National School Lunch Program? What is there to stop coalitions of concerned parents from taking those discussions to local school board meetings? What is there to stop proud local communities from engaging these issues? These are political concerns that affect everyone in our society. I do not mean the politics-as-spectacle that we sometimes see on traditional TV news, but politics-as-personal. Politics as a struggle for survival.

I recognize that some will dismiss these goals as pie-in-the-sky utopianism. Surely the communication among large groups of people is a far clumsier negotiation than the almost instantaneous intracellular communication described above. Although that may be true to a certain extent, this is exactly what the current power structure would have you believe. I am not so cynical. We are our own greatest impediment to meaningful change, on both an individual and collective level, but we are also our own greatest opportunity.

Whatever the difficulties, I do not believe that we should abandon Nature's guiding principles. Besides, we're already closer to Nature's model than many of the naysayers may realize, for all of us are bound together by a tangible substance: food. Though we have constructed degrees of separation between ourselves and food by entrusting the practice of agriculture and food production to a shrinking minority of corporations, we will never be free from its grip. *Food is of universal interest.* Through the biochemical exchange of energy, from the sun to plants, from plants to animals, and from animals to other animals, we all sup from the same malleable energy trough. Food is merely the temporary vehicle for transport and distribution of that energy, and the determination of which energy sources we should consume is of universal importance.

My suggestion that we "cut out the middle livestock" and go straight for the energy provided by plants is based on a wholistic understanding of the science of nutrition. Nutrition, as a concept, appeals to a narrower subset of people than food; it carries a more sterile and intimidating set of connotations (perhaps this is why there's no Nutrition Network to compete with the Food Network). However, that does not make nutrition's impact any less universal than food's. We must not forget: nutrition is food in action. And the replicable evidence on the activities of food's nutrient parts, including the biological pathways that interconnect these parts with one another and with the outside world of observable effects, offers unambiguous proof that *our subsistence is wedded to Nature's wholism.* And if our subsistence is wedded to Nature's wholism, then Nature is an essentially personal, societal, and moral concern. If Nature is potent, then so are we. Perhaps we have forgotten how to utilize that strength, but that does not mean it is lost to us forever.

And so, yes—moving forward, I call for the acceptance and celebration of our personal stake in Nature. For recognition of our integration and interdependence, which is more profound than we can communicate within the strictures of language. In the present age of earnest myopia and opportunistic reductionism, this recognition offers a radical alternative. It says that beneath the hubbub of modern life, between all the layers of illusion and separation that we construct and imagine, *we are actual miracles of biology.*

I will not speculate about why we became so convinced of our separation from Nature, but we must admit that the illusion exists. Elsewhere in nature, we do not see animals so devastatingly imbalanced as we have become. We do not see "health" stores and weight-loss centers nestled in the branches of every other oak and willow. Though disease and destruction exist in the rest of the natural world, they are many orders of magnitude less severe than the disease and destruction caused by humankind. And when we investigate the origin of these complications, we discover even more the means by which Nature restores and maintains balance. We discover natural mechanisms, such as fasting, by which the creatures of nature restore health. What we do not see are other creatures turning to isolated, synthetic reproductions of Nature in order to survive (this is what all drugs are: isolated, synthetic reproductions of natural compounds). Other creatures do not wage ineffective "wars on cancer" (and especially not while simultaneously behaving in ways that increase the likelihood of developing cancer). They do not organize into "national institutes" to address problems of their own creation. They do not fall prey to the marketing machines that sell short-term effects without regard for long-term health. As far as I know, other creatures do not celebrate their ingenuity as much as we do, but neither do they need to. Instead, they express inborn wisdom.

We have inborn wisdom, too. If we can accept that, and act in accordance with our miraculous Nature—if we behave as if Nature depends on our behavior, for it does; if we eat as if Nature depends on our eating, for it does; and if we organize as if part of a whole, for we are—there may yet be a future for us all. Nature is prepared for that future. Might we go along for the ride?

NOTES

Preface and Acknowledgments

1   Yzaguirre, M. R. The decline of university tenure makes it harder to defend politically. *The Hill.* (2017). https://thehill.com/blogs/pundits-blog/education/319979-the-decline-of-university -tenure-makes-it-harder-to-defend.

Introduction

1   US Senate, Select Committee on Nutrition and Human Needs. *Dietary goals for the United States,* 2nd ed. (US Government Printing Office, 1977), 83.

2   National Research Council. *Recommended dietary allowances,* 9th ed. (National Academies Press, 1980).

3   Committee on Diet, Nutrition, and Cancer. *Diet, nutrition and cancer.* (National Academies Press, 1982).

4   Committee on Diet, Nutrition, and Cancer. *Diet, nutrition and cancer: Directions for research.* (National Academies Press, 1983).

5   Jukes, T. H. *The day that food was declared a poison.* 42-45 (Council for Agricultural Science and Technology, Ames, IO, 1982).

6   Garst, J. E. *Comments on diet, nutrition and cancer.* 28–29 (Ames, IA, 1982).

Chapter One

1   Nichols, H. What are the leading causes of death in the US? *Medical News Today* (2019). https://www.medicalnewstoday.com/articles/282929.php.

2   Esselstyn, C. B., Jr., Gendy, G., Doyle, J., Golubic, M., & Roizen, M. F. A way to reverse CAD? *J Fam. Pract.* 63, 356–364b (2014).

3   Doll, R. & Peto, R. The causes of cancer: quantitative estimates of avoidable risks of cancer in the United States today. *J Natl Cancer Inst* 66, 1191–1308 (1981).

4   Statista. *Global pharmaceutical industry—statistics and facts* (2017). https://www.statista.com/topics /1764/global-pharmaceutical-industry/.

5   Preidt, R. Americans taking more prescription drugs than ever. *WebMD* (2017). https://www. webmd.com/drug-medication/news/20170803/americans-taking-more-prescription-drugs-than -ever-survey.

6   Fuller, P. Kiwi doctors lobby for crackdown on drug ads. *Stuff* (2018). https://www.stuff.co.nz/ national/health/107546694/advertising-prescription-drugs-should-it-be-allowed-in-nz.

7   Amadeo, K. The rising cost of health care by year and its causes. *The Balance* (2019). https://www
.thebalance.com/causes-of-rising-healthcare-costs-4064878.

8   Kane, J. Health care costs: how the U.S. compares with other countries. *PBS NewsHour* (2012).
https://www.pbs.org/newshour/health/health-costs-how-the-us-compares-with-other-countries.

9   World Health Organization. *Diet, nutrition and the prevention of chronic diseases. Report of a Joint
WHO/FAO Expert Consultation.* (World Health Organization, 2003).

10   Crimmins, E. M. & Beltran-Sanchez, H. Mortality and morbidity trends: is there compression of
morbidity? *J Gerontol B Psychol Sci Soc Sci* 66, 75–86, doi:10.1093/geronb/gbq088 (2011).

11   Hanowell, B. Life expectancy is, overall, increasing. *SlateGroup* (2016). https://slate.com
/technology/2016/12/life-expectancy-is-still-increasing.html.

12   Solly, M. U.S. life expectancy drops for third year in a row, reflecting rising drug overdoses, suicides.
Smart News (2018). https://www.smithsonianmag.com/smart-news/us-life-expectancy-drops-third
-year-row-reflecting-rising-drug-overdose-suicide-rates-180970942/.

13   Redfield, R. R. *CDC director's media statement on US life expectancy.* (US Department of Health and
Human Services, CDC Newsroom, 2018). https://www.cdc.gov/media/releases/2018/s1129-US-
life-expectancy.html

14   Himmelstein, D. E., Warren, E., Thorne, D., & Woolhander, S. Illness and injury as contributors
to bankruptcy. *Health Affairs Web Exclusive* W5–63 (2009).

15   Avalere Health LLC. *Total cost of cancer care by site of service: physician office vs outpatient hospital*
(2012). http://www.communityoncology.org/pdfs/avalere-cost-of-cancer-care-study.pdf.

16   Beltran-Sanchez, H., Preston, S. H., & Canudas-Romo, V. An integrated approach to cause-of-
death analysis: cause-deleted life tables and decompositions of life expectancy. *Demogr Res* 19,
1323, doi:10.4054/DemRes.2008.19.35 (2008).

17   Vallin, J. & Mesle, F. The segmented trend line of highest life expectancies. *Pop. Develop. Rev.* 35
159–187, http://www.jstor.org/stable/25487645 (2009).

18   Kamal, R., Cox, C., & McDermott, D. What Are the Recent and Forecasted Trends in Prescription Drug Spending? Growth in Prescription Spending Has Slowed Again in 2017, after
Increasing Rapidly in 2014 and 2015. *Peterson-KFF Health System Tracker* (2019). https://www.
healthsystemtracker.org/chart-collection/recent-forecasted-trends-prescription-drug-spending
/#item-start.

19   Light, D. W. New prescription drugs: a major health risk with few offsetting advantages. (2014).
https://ethics.harvard.edu/blog/new-prescription-drugs-major-health-risk-few-offsetting
-advantages.

20   Public Citizen's Health Research Group. Worst pills, best pills. An expert, independent second
opinion on more than 1,800 prescription drugs, over-the-counter medications and supplements
(2019). https://www.worstpills.org/public/page.cfm?op_id=4.

21   Starfield, B. *Primary care: balancing health needs, services, and technology* (Oxford University Press,
1998).

22   US Food & Drug Administration. Preventable adverse drug reactions: a focus on drug interactions.
(2018). https://www.fda.gov/drugs/drug-interactions-labeling/preventable-adverse-drug-reactions
-focus-drug-interactions.

23   Kaiser Family Foundation. *Total health care employment.* (2017). https://www.kff.org/other/state
-indicator/total-health-care-employment/?currentTimeframe=0&sortModel=%7B%22colId%22:
%22Location%22,%22sort%22:%22asc%22%7D.

24   World Population Review. Life expectancy by country 2017 (2017). http://worldpopulationreview
.com/countries/life-expectancy-by-country/.

25   Mikulic, M. Global pharmaceutical industry—statistics and facts. *Statista* (2019). https://www
.statista.com/topics/1764/global-pharmaceutical-industry/.

26   Wikipedia. List of countries by government budget. *Wikipedia* (2019). https://en.wikipedia.org
/wiki/List_of_countries_by_government_budget.

27   Kannel, W. B., Dawber, T. R., Kagan, A., Revotskie, N., & Stokes, J. Factors of risk in the development of coronary heart disease—six-year follow-up experience. *Ann. Internal Medi.* 55, 33–50 (1961).

28   Jolliffe, N. & Archer, M. Statistical associations between international coronary heart disease death rates and certain environmental factors. *J. Chronic Dis.* 9, 636–652 (1959).

29   Stemmermann, G. N., Nomura, A. M. Y., Heilbrun, L. K., Pollack, E. S., & Kagan, A. Serum cholesterol and colon cancer incidence in Hawaiian Japanese men. *J. Natl. Cancer Inst.* 67, 1179–1182 (1981).

30   Kagan, A., Harris, B. R., & Winkelstein, W. Epidemiologic studies of coronary heart disease and stroke in Japanese men living in Japan, Hawaii and California. *J. Chronic Dis.* 27, 345–364 (1974).

31   Kato, H., Tillotson, J., Nichaman, M. Z., Rhoads, G., & Hamilton, H. B. Epidemiologic studies of coronary heart disease and stroke in Japanese men living in Japan, Hawaii and California: serum lipids and diet. *Am. J. Epidemiol.* 97, 372–385 (1973).

32   Morrison, L. M. Arteriosclerosis. *JAMA* 145, 1232–1236 (1951).

33   Ornish, D., Brown, S. E., Scherwitz, L. W., Billings, J. H., Armstrong, W. T., Ports, T. A. et al. Can lifestyle changes reverse coronary heart disease? *Lancet* 336, 129–133 (1990).

34   Sipherd, R. The third-leading cause of death in US most doctors don't want you to know about. *CNBC* (2018). https://www.cnbc.com/2018/02/22/medical-errors-third-leading-cause-of-death -in-america.html.

35   Scrimgeour, E. M., McCall, M. G., Smith, D. E., & Masarei, J. R. L. Levels of serum cholesterol, triglyceride, HDL cholesterol, apolipoproteins A-1 and B, and plasma glucose, and prevalence of diastolic hypertension and cigarette smoking in Papua New Guinea Highlanders. *Pathology* 21, 46–50 (1989).

36   National Cancer Institute. National Cancer Act of 1971 (2016). https://www.cancer.gov/ about-nci/legislative/history/national-cancer-act-1971#declarations.

37   Hanahan, D. Rethinking the war on cancer. *Lancet* 383, 558-563, doi:10.1016/S0140-6736(13) 62226-6 (2014).

38   Vineis, P. & Wild, C. P. Global cancer patterns: causes and prevention. *Lancet* 383, 549-557, doi:10.1016/S0140-6736(13)62224-2 (2014).

Chapter Two

1   Slonaker, J. R. The effect of different percents of protein in the diet. VII. Life span and cause of death. *Am. J. Physiol.* 98, 266–275 (1931).

2   Hoffman, F. L. *Cancer and diet.* (Williams and Wilkins Co., 1937).

3   Sypher, F. J. The rediscovered prophet: Frederick L. Hoffman (1865–1946). *The Cosmos Journal* (2012).

4   Anonymous. Frederick L. Hoffman. In *Who Was Who in America* Vol. 2 (Marquis Who's Who, Inc., Chicago IL, 1943–1950).

5   Cassedy, J. H. Hoffman, Frederick Ludwig. *DAB Suppl. 4* (1946–1950).

6   Hoffman, F. L. San Francisco survey. Preliminary and final reports. (Prudential Press, 1924–1934).

7   Hoffman, F. L. *The mortality from throughout the world.* (The Prudential Press, 1915).

8   Hoffman, F. L. The menace of cancer. *Trans. Amer. Gynecological Soc* 38, 397–452 (1913).

9   American Cancer Society. Minutes of National Council Meeting (Friday, May 6, 1921), campaign notes, No. 3 (1921). Cited in Triolo, V. A. & Shimkin, M. B. The American Cancer Society and cancer research origins and organization: 1913–1943. *Cancer Res.* 29, 1615–1641 (1969).

10   Hoffman, F. L., Cancer and Smoking Habits, in *Cancer* (ed. F. E. Adair), 50–67 (J. B. Lippincott Co, 1931).

11   Wynder, E. L. & Graham, E. A. Tobacco smoking as possible etiologic factor in bronchiogenic carcinoma: study of 684 proved cases. *JAMA* 143, 329–336 (1950).

12   Doll, R. & Hill, A. B. A study of the aetiology of carcinoma of the lung. *Brit. Med. J.* 2, 1271–1286 (1952).

13   US Public Health Service. *Smoking and health.* (Washington, DC: US Government Printing Office, 1964).

14   Deelman, H. J., in *International symposium, American Society for the Control of Cancer* (Lake Mohonk, NY, 1926).

15   Bashford, E. F. Fresh alarms on the increase of cancer. *Lancet*, 319–382 (1914).

16   Austoker, J. The "treatment of choice": breast cancer surgery 1860–1985. *Soc. Soc. Hist. Med. Bull. (London)* 37, 100–107 (1985).

17   Hayward, J. The principles of conservative treatment for early breast cancer. *Handlinger* 141, 168–171 (1981).

18   Hoffman, F. L. Fallacies of birth control, in *Delaware Medical Society* (Dover, Delaware, 1926).

19   Hoffman, F. L. "The Menace to Cancer" and American vital statistics. *Lancet*, 1079–1083 (1914).

20   Hoffman, F. L., in *Jubliee Historical Volume of the American Public Health Association* (ed. M. P. Ravenel), 94–117 (1921).

21   Hoffman, F. L. National health insurance and the medical profession, (1920).

22   Rosen, G. *A history of public health: MD monographs on medical history*, Vol. 1. (MD Publications, 1958).

23   Hoffman, F. L. The mortality from consumption to the dusty trade. *US Bureau of Labor Bulletin No. 79* (Washington DC, 1908).

24   Hoffman, F. L. in *Fifth Annual Welfare and Efficiency Conference* (Harrisburg, PA, 1917).

25   Cameron, V. & Long, E. R. Tuberculosis medical research. (1959).

26   Triolo, V. A. & Riegel, I. L. The American Association for Cancer Research, 1907–1940. Historical review. *Cancer Res.* 21, 137–167 (1961).

27   Rigney, E. H. The American Society for the Control of Cancer, 1913–1943. (New York City Cancer Committee Publ., 1944).

28   British Empire Cancer Campaign. Notes on cancer. (Chorley & Pickersgill, Ltd., 1923).

29   Lakeman, C. E. Cancer as a public health problem (cited in Triolo and Shimkin, 1969). (1914).

30   Handley, W. S. *The genesis and prevention of cancer.* (John Murray, 1955).

31   Soper, G. A. A recent English opinion on cancer. A review of a series of lectures delivered under the auspices of the Fellowship of Medicine, London, 1925. (American Society for the Control of Cancer, 1926).

32   Soper, G. A., in *International symposium, American Society for the Control of Cancer,* 148–154 (Lake Mohonk, NY, 1926).

33   Lilienthal, H., in *International symposium,* 308–317.

34   Handley, W. S., in *International symposium,* 22–30.

35   Hoffman, F. L. Personal lecture: On the causation of cancer. April 17, 1924, in *American Association for Cancer Research* (Buffalo, NY, 1924).

36   Hoffman, F. L. Radium (mesothorium) necrosis. *JAMA* 85, 961–965 (1925).

37   Hoffman, F. L. Personal lecture: Cancer in Mexico, in *American Association for Cancer Research Meetings* (Rochester, NY, 1927).

38   Lambe, W. *Reports on the effects of a peculiar regimen on scirrhous tumors and cancerous ulcers.* (J. M'Creary, 1809).

39   Celsus. *de Celsus Medicina.* Cited by Lambe, W. *Additional reports on the effects of a peculiar regimen in cases of cancer, scrofula, consumption, asthma, and other chronic diseases.* (J. Mawman, 1815).

40   Erasmus, W. *The history of Middlesex Hospital.* (John Churchill, 1845). Ch. 137–144.

41   Spencer, C. *Vegetarianism, a history.* (Four Walls Eight Windows, 1993).

42   Bennett, J. H. *On cancerous and cancroid growths.* (Sutherland and Knox, 1849).

43   Bennett, J. H. *Clinical lectures on the principles and practice of medicine,* 4th ed. (Adam and Charles Black, 1865).

44   MacIlwain, G. *The general nature and treatment of tumors.* (John Churchill, 1845).

45   Shaw, J. *The cure of cancer: and how surgery blocks the way.* (F. S. Turney, 1907).

46   Walshe, W. H. *The nature and treatment of cancer.* (Taylor and Walton, 1846).

47   Howard, J. *Practical observations on cancer.* (J. Hatchard, 1811).

48 Thomson, W. B. *Cancer: is it preventable?* (Chatto and Winders, 1932).
49 Burkitt, D. P. & Trowell, H. C. *Refined carbohydrate foods and disease: some implications of dietary fibre.* (Academic Press, 1975).
50 Braithwaite, J., in *What is the root cause of cancer* (ed. F. T. Marwood). 27–31 (John Bale, Sons and Danielson, Ltd., 1924).
51 Hare, F. *The food factor in disease.* Vol. II (Longmans, Green and Company, 1905).
52 Williams, W. R. *The natural history of cancer, with special references to its causation and prevention.* (William Heinemann, 1908).
53 Lambe, W. *Additional reports on the effects of a peculiar regimen in cases of cancer, scrofula, consumption, asthma, and other chronic diseases.* (J. Mawman, 1815).
54 Li, J.-Y. Epidemiology of esophageal cancer in China. *Natl. Cancer Inst. Monograph* 62, 113–120 (1982).
55 Wiseman, R. *Several Chirurgicall Treatises.* (E. Flesher and J. Macock, 1676).

Chapter Three

1   MacIlwain, G. *The general nature and treatment of tumors.* (John Churchill, 1845).
2   MacIlwain, G. *Memoirs of John Abernethy, F.R.S., with a view of his lectures, writings and character.* (Harper & Brothers, 1853).
3   Rabagliati, A. *The causes of cancer and the means to be adopted for its prevention.* (C. W. Daniel Company, 1924).
4   Russell, R. *Preventable cancer. Statistical research.* (Longmans, Green and Co., 1912).
5   Thomson, W. B. *Cancer: is it preventable?* (Chatto and Winders, 1932).
6   Williams, W. R. *The principles of cancer and tumor formation.* (John Bale and Sons, 1888).
7   Barker, J. E. *Cancer, how it is caused: how it can be prevented. Introduced by Sir W. Arbuthnot Lane.* (Murray, 1924).
8   Russell, F. A. R. The reduction of cancer. (1907). Franklin Classics.
9   Campbell, T. C. Cancer prevention and treatment by wholistic nutrition. *J. Nat. Sci.* Oct 3, e448 (2017).
10 Hoffman, F. L. *Cancer and diet.* (Williams and Wilkins Co., 1937).
11 Bulkley, L. D. *Cancer and its non-surgical treatment.* (1921). William Wood & Co.
12 Hoffman, F. L., in *The Belgian National Cancer Congress.* Brussels, Belgium, Conf. Proceedings.
13 Hoffman, F. L. Personal lecture: On the causation of cancer. April 17, 1924, in *American Association for Cancer Research* (Buffalo, NY, 1924).
14 Hoffman, F. L. San Francisco survey. Preliminary and final reports. (Prudential Press, 1924–1934).
15 Williams, W. R. *The natural history of cancer, with special references to its causation and prevention.* (William Heinemann, 1908).
16 Bell, B. *A system of surgery* (Elliot, C., 1784). Cited in Williams, W. R. *The principles of cancer and tumor formation.* (John Bale and Sons, 1888).
17 Lambe, W. *Reports on the effects of a peculiar regimen on scirrhous tumors and cancerous ulcers.* (J. M'Creary, 1809).
18 Lambe, W. *Additional reports on the effects of a peculiar regimen in cases of cancer, scrofula, consumption, asthma, and other chronic diseases.* (J. Mawman, 1815).
19 Howard, J. *Practical observations on cancer.* (J. Hatchard, 1811).
20 Bennett, J. H. *On cancerous and cancroid growths.* (Sutherland and Knox, 1849).
21 Jenner, W. Discussion on cancer (in chair). *Trans. Path. Soc. (London)* 25, 289–402 (1873–1874).
22 Mitchell, R. *A general and historical treatise on cancer life: its causes, progress, and treatment.* (J&A Churchill, 1879).
23 Bulkley, L. D. *Cancer, its cause and treatment.* (Paul B. Hoeber, 1917).
24 Triolo, V. A. & Riegel, I. L. The American Association for Cancer Research, 1907–1940. Historical review. *Cancer Res.* 21, 137–167 (1961).

25   Austoker, J. The "treatment of choice": breast cancer surgery 1860–1985. *Soc. Soc. Hist. Med. Bull. (London)* 37, 100–107 (1985).

26   Shimkin, M. B. Thirteen questions: some historical outlines for cancer research. *J. Natl. Cancer Inst.* 19, 307–314 (1957).

27   Bainbridge, W. S. *The cancer problem.* (Macmillan Co., 1914).

28   Triolo, V. A. & Shimkin, M. B. The American Cancer Society and cancer research origins and organization: 1913–1943. *Cancer Res.* 29, 1615–1641 (1969).

29   Gibson, C. L. Final results in the surgery of malignant disease. *Ann. Surg.* 84, 158–173 (1926).

30   Lakeman, C. E. Cancer as a public health problem. (1914). Cited in Triolo, V. A. & Shimkin, M. B. The American Cancer Society and cancer research origins and organization: 1913–1943. *Cancer Res.* 29, 1615–1641 (1969).

31   American Cancer Society. Minutes of National Council Meeting (Friday, May 6, 1921), campaign notes, No. 3. (1921). Cited in Triolo, V. A. & Shimkin, M. B. The American Cancer Society and cancer research origins and organization: 1913–1943. *Cancer Res.* 29, 1615–1641 (1969).

32   Soper, G. A. A recent English opinion on cancer. A review of a series of lectures delivered under the auspices of the Fellowship of Medicine, London, 1925. (American Society for the Control of Cancer, 1926).

33   Hoffman, F. L. Radium (mesothorium) necrosis. *JAMA* 85, 961–965 (1925).

34   Castle, W. B., Drinker, K. R. & Drinker, C. K. Necrosis of the jaw in workers employed in applying a luminous paint containing radium. *J. Ind. Hyg.* 7, 371–382 (1925).

35   Hartland, H. S., Conlon, P., & Knef, J. P. Some unrecognized dangers in the use of handling of radioactive substances: with special reference to the storage of unsoluble products of radium and mesothorium in the reticulo-endothelial system. *JAMA* 85, 1769–1776 (1925).

36   Wood, F. C. Demonstration of the methods and results of cancer research. *Campaign Notes* 10 (1928).

37   Copeman, S. M. & Greenwood, M. Diet and cancer, with special reference to the incidence of cancer upon members of certain religious orders. (Ministry of Health, His Majesty's Stationery Office, London, 1926).

38   Wood, F. C., in *International symposium,* 318–325 (Lake Mohonk, NY, 1926).

39   Delbert, P. Tentatives de traitement de cancer par le selenium. *Bull. de l'assoc. franc. pur l'etude du cancer (Paris),* 121–125 (1912).

40   Blumenthal, A. De la reaction febrile consecutive aux injection intra-veineuses de selenium colloidale. *Portou Med. Pontiers* 28, 238 (1913).

41   Anonymous. Groundless fear of radium. *Campaign Notes* 10 (1936).

42   Cramer, W. & Horning, E. S. Experimental production by oestrin of pituitary tumors. *Bulletin* 18 (1936).

43   Moschcowitz, A. V., Colp, R., & Klingenstein, P. Late results after amputation of the breast. *Ann. Surg.* 84, 174–184 (1926).

44   Bulkley, L. D. Precancerous conditions. *Interstate Med. Journ.,* 730–734.

45   Lilienthal, H. in *American Society for the Control of Cancer.* 308–317.

46   Bell, Robert. *Ten years' record of the treatment of cancer without operation.* (Dean and Son, Ltd., 1906).

47   Shaw, J. *The cure of cancer: and how surgery blocks the way.* (F. S. Turney, 1907).

48   Cairns, J. The history of mortality and the conquest of cancer. *Accomplishments in Cancer Research,* 90–105 (1985).

49   Bailar, J. C. & Smith, E. M. Progress against cancer? *New Engl. J. Med.* 314, 1226–1232 (1986).

50   Sweet, J. E., Corson-White, E. P., & Saxon, G. J. The relation of diets and of castration to the transmissible tumors of rats and mice. *J. Biol. Chem.* 15, 181–191 (1913).

51   Rous, P. The influence of diet on transplanted and spontaneous mouse tumors. *J. Exp. Med.* 20, 433–451 (1914).

52   Hoffman, F. L. The menace of cancer. *Trans. Amer. Gynecological Soc* 38, 397–452 (1913).

53   Rigney, E. H. *The American Society for the Control of Cancer, 1913–1943.* (New York: New York City Cancer Committee Publ., 1944).

54   Bashford, E. F. Fresh alarms on the increase of cancer. *Lancet*, 319–382 (1914).

55   Austoker, J. The politics of cancer research: Walter Morley Fletcher and the origins of the British Empire cancer campaign. *Soc. Soc. Hist. Med. Bull. (Lond.)* 37, 63–67 (1985).

56   British Empire Cancer Campaign. *The truth about cancer.* (John Murray, 1930).

57   Lockhart-Mummery, J.P. *The origin of cancer.* (J&A Churchill, 1934).

58   British Empire Cancer Campaign. Series of annual reports. (London: British Empire Cancer Campaign, 1923–1934).

59   Hoffman, F. L., in *American Society for the Control of Cancer.* (American Society for the Control of Cancer, 1928).

60   Childe, C. P. President's address on environment and health. Ninety-first annual meeting of British Medical Associaton. *Brit. Med. J.*, 135–140 (1923).

61   Handley, W. S. *Cancer research at the Middlesex Hospital, 1900–1924.* (London, 1924).

62   Austoker, J. The origins of cancer research, 1802–1902. (Wellcome Unit for the History of Medicine, 1985).

63   Halstead, W. S. The results of radical operations for the cure of carcinoma of the breast. *Ann. Surgery* 46, 1–19 (1907).

64   Handley, W. S. *The genesis of cancer.* (Kegan Paul, Trench, Trubner & Co., Ltd., 1931).

65   Handley, W. S. *The genesis and prevention of cancer.* (John Murray, 1955).

66   Bayly, M. B. *Cancer: the failure of modern research. A survey.* (The Health Education and Research Council, 1936).

67   Clowes, G. H. A. A study of the influence exerted by a variety of physical and chemical forces on the virulence of carcinoma in mice and of the conditions under which immunity against cancer may be experimentally induced in these animals. *Brit. Med. J.*, 1548–1554 (1906).

68   Hoffman, F. L. "The Menace to Cancer" and American vital statistics. *Lancet*, 1079–1083 (1914).

69   Adair, F. E., in *International contributions to the study of cancer in honor of James Ewing* (ed. F. E. Adair), editorial comments, (J. B. Lippincott Co., 1931).

70   Welche, W. H., in *International contributions to the study of cancer in honor of James Ewing* (ed. F. E. Adair), (J.B. Lippincott Co., 1931).

71   Ewing, J. The prevention of cancer, in *American Society for the Control of Cancer* (Lake Mohonk, NY, 1926).

72   Erasmus, W. *The history of Middlesex Hospital.* (John Churchill, 1845). Ch. 137–144.

73   Campbell, T. C. Chemical carcinogens and human risk assessment. *Fed. Proc.* 39, 2467–2484 (1980).

74   Avalere Health LLC. *Total cost of cancer care by site of service: physician office vs. outpatient hospital* (2012). http://www.communityoncology.org/pdfs/avalere-cost-of-cancer-care-study.pdf.

75   Morgan, G., Ward, R., & Barton, M. The contribution of cytotoxic chemotherapy to 5-year survival in adult malignancies. *Clin. Oncol. (R. Coll. Radiol.)* 16, 549–560 (2004).

76   Kagan, J. European Medicines Agency (EMA). *Investopedia* (2019). https://www.investopedia.com/terms/e/european-medicines-agency-ema.asp.

77   Home Precautions After Chemotherapy. *Roswellpark.org* (2020). https://www.roswellpark.org/cancer-care/treatments/cancer-drugs/post-chemo-guide.

Chapter Four

1   Campbell, T. C. Nutrition renaissance and public health policy. *J. Nutr. Biology* 3, 124–138, doi:10.1080/01635581.2017.1339094 (2017).

2   Press release, National Academy of Sciences, (ed. The National Academies). (National Research Council, Institute of Medicine, Washington, DC, 2002).

3   Wikipedia. *Nestlé.* (2018). https://en.wikipedia.org/wiki/Nestl%C3%A9.

4   Sharma, S., Dortch, K. S., Byrd-Williams, C., Truxillio, J. B., Rahman, G. A., Bonsu, P. et al. Nutrition-related knowledge, attitudes, and dietary behaviors among Head Start teachers in Texas: a cross-sectional study. *J. Acad. Nutr. Diet* 113, 558–562, doi:10.1016/j.jand.2013.01.003 (2013).

5   Hoek, J. Informed choice and the nanny state: learning from the tobacco industry. *Public Health* 129, 1038–1045, doi:10.1016/j.puhe.2015.03.009 (2015).

Chapter Five

1   The paper where Mulder named protein, according to Munro (1964), is Mulder, G. J., *J. Prakt. Chem.* 16, 29 (1839).

2   Mulder, G. J. *The chemistry of vegetable & animal physiology* (trans. P. F. H. Fromberg). (W. Blackwood & Sons, 1849).

3   Munro, H. N., in *Mammalian protein metabolism*, Vol. I (eds. H. N. Munro & J. B. Allison), 1–29 (Academic Press, 1964).

4   Lewis, H. B., in *Mammalian protein metabolism*, Vol. I (eds. H. N. Munro & J. B. Allison), 13–32 (Academic Press, 1964).

5   Voit, C. Ueber die kost eines vegetariers. *Zeitschr. f. Biologie* 25, 261 (1889). Cited by Chittenden, R. H. *Physiological economy in nutrition*. (F.A. Stokes, 1904), 5.

6   Chittenden, R. H. *Physiological economy in nutrition*. (F.A. Stokes, 1904).

7   Spencer, C. *Vegetarianism, a History*. (Four Walls Eight Windows, 1993).

8   Mitchell, H. H. Does a Low-Protein Diet Produce Racial Inferiority? *Science, New Series* 38, no. 970, 156–58 (1913).

9   Agriculture Research Service. *History of human nutrition research in the U.S. Department of Agriculture, Agricultural Research Service: people, events, and accomplishments* (United States Department of Agriculture, Agriculture Research Service, 2017), 356.

10   Mitchell, H. H. A method of determining the biological value of protein. *J. Biol. Chem.* 58, 873–903 (1924).

11   Sarwar, G. & McDonough, F. E. Evaluation of protein digestibility-corrected amino acid score method for assessing protein quality of foods. *J. Assoc. of Anal. Chem.* 73, 347–356 (1990).

12   Key, T. J. A., Chen, J., Wang, D. Y., Pike, M. C., & Boreham, J. Sex hormones in women in rural China and in Britain. *Brit. J. Cancer* 62, 631–636 (1990).

13   Marshall, J. R., Qu, Y., Chen, J., Parpia, B., & Campbell, T. C. Additional ecologic evidence: lipids and breast cancer mortality among women age 55 and over in China. *Europ. J. Cancer* 28A, 1720–1727 (1991).

14   Chen, J., Campbell, T. C., Li, J., & Peto, R. *Diet, life-style and mortality in China. A study of the characteristics of 65 Chinese counties.* (Oxford University Press; Cornell University Press; People's Medical Publishing House, 1990).

15   Grant, W. B. An ecologic study of dietary links to prostate cancer. *Altern. Med. Rev.* 4, 162–169 (1999).

16   Giles, G. G., Severi, G., English, D. R., McCredie, M. R., MacInnis, R., Boyle, P. et al. Early growth, adult body size and prostate cancer risk. *Int. J. Cancer* 103, 241–245, doi:10.1002/ijc.10810 (2003).

17   Pike, M. C., Spicer, D. V., Dahmoush, L., & Press, M. F. Estrogens, progestogens, normal breast cell proliferation, and breast cancer risk. *Epidemiol. Revs.* 15, 17–35 (1993).

18   Cheng, Z., Hu, J., King, J., Jay, G., & Campbell, T. C. Inhibition of hepatocellular carcinoma development in hepatitis B virus transfected mice by low dietary casein. *Hepatology* 26, 1351–1354 (1997).

19   Hu, J., Chisari, F. V., & Campbell, T. C. Modulating effect of dietary protein on transgene expression in hepatitis B virus (HBV) transgenic mice. *Cancer Research* 35, 104 Abs. (1994).

20   Schulsinger, D. A., Root, M. M., & Campbell, T. C. Effect of dietary protein quality on development of aflatoxin B1-induced hepatic preneoplastic lesions. *J. Natl. Cancer Inst.* 81, 1241–1245 (1989).

21 Burkitt, D. P. Epidemiology of cancer of the colon and the rectum. *Cancer* 28, 3–13 (1971).

22 Drasar, B. S. & Irving, D. Environmental factors and cancer of the colon and breast. *Br. J. Cancer* 27, 167–172 (1973).

23 Reddy, B. S. & Wynder, E. L. Large bowel carcinogenesis: fecal constituents of populations with disease incidence rates of colon cancer. *J. Nat. Cancer Inst.* 50, 1437–1442 (1973).

24 Mafra, D., Borges, N. A., Cardozo, L., Anjos, J. S., Black, A. P., Moraes, C., et al. Red meat intake in chronic kidney disease patients: two sides of the coin. *Nutrition* 46, 26–32, doi:10.1016/j.nut.2017.08.015 (2018).

25 Campbell, T. M. & Liebman, S. E. Plant-based dietary approach to stage 3 chronic kidney disease with hyperphosphatemia. *Brit. Med. J. Case Rept.* 12:e:e232080, doi:10.1136/bcr-2019-232080 (2019).

26 Rhee, C. M., Ahmadi, S. F., Kovesdy, C. P., & Kalantar-Zadeh, K. Low-protein diet for conservative management of chronic kidney disease: a systematic review and meta-analysis of controlled trials. *J. Cachexia Sarcopenia Muscle* 9, 235–245, doi:10.1002/jcsm.12264 (2018).

27 Bikbov, B., Perico, N., & Remuzzi, G., on behalf of the GBD Genitourinary Diseases Expert Group. Disparities in chronic kidney disease prevalence among males and females in 195 countries: analysis of the Global Burden of Disease 2016 Study. *Nephron* 139, 313–318, doi:10.1159/000489897 (2018).

28 Williams, C. D. A nutritional disease of childhood associated with a maize diet. *Arch. Dis. Child.* 8, 423–433 (1933).

29 Agarwal, K. N., Bhatia, B. D., Agarwal, D. K., & Shankar, R. Assessment of protein energy needs of Indian adults using short-term nitrogen balance methodolgy: protein-energy-requirement studies in developing countries: results of international research, in *Food and Nutrition Bulletin Supplement* 10 (eds. W. M. Rand, R. Uauy, & N. S. Scrimshaw), 89–95 (The United Nations University, 1983).

30 Scrimshaw, N. S. History and early development of INCAP. *J. Nutr.* 140, 394–396, doi:10.3945/jn.109.114694 (2010).

31 Waterlow, J. C. & Payne, P. R. The protein gap. *Nature* 258, 113–117 (1975).

32 McLaren, D. S. The great protein fiasco. *Lancet* July 13, 1974, 93–96 (1974).

33 Bressani, R. INCAP studies of vegetable proteins for human consumption. *Food Nutr. Bull.* 31, 95–110, doi:10.1177/156482651003100110 (2010).

34 Scrimshaw, N. S. Iron deficiency. *Sci. Amer.* October, 46–52 (1991).

35 Lancaster, M. C., Jenkins, F. P., & Philp, J. M. Toxicity associated with certain samples of groundnuts. *Nature* 192, 1095–1096 (1961).

36 Campbell, T. C., Caedo, J. P., Jr., Bulatao-Jayme, J., Salamat, L., & Engel, R. W. Aflatoxin M_1 in human urine. *Nature* 227, 403–404 (1970).

37 Campbell, T. C. & Salamat, L. A., in *Mycotoxins in human health* (ed. I. F. Purchase), 263–269 (Macmillan, 1971).

38 Campbell, T. C. & Stoloff, L. Implications of mycotoxins for human health. *J. Agr. Food Chem.* 22, 1006–1015 (1974).

39 Merrill, A. H., Jr. & Campbell, T. C. Preliminary study of in vitro aflatoxin B_1 metabolism by human liver. *J. Tox. Appl. Pharmacol.* 27, 210–213 (1973).

40 Chittenden, R. H. *The nutrition of man.* (F. A. Stokes & Co., 1907).

41 Fisher, I. *The influence of flesh-eating on endurance.* (Modern Medicine Publishing, 1908).

42 Asp, K. Vegan in the NFL: how 15 Tennessee Titans made the switch. (2018). https://www.forksoverknives.com/tennessee-titans-nfl-teams-shift-veganism/#gs.v_FW3Ho.

43 Hinds, J. *Monkeybar Gym–Madison*, https://www.linkedin.com/company/monkey-bar-gym---madison/about/ (2000).

44 Campbell, T. C. Addendum to Spock, B. Why parents should keep children meat and dairy free. *New Century Newsletter* (1997). https://nutritionstudies.org/why-parents-should-keep-children-meat-and-dairy-free/.

45 Wikipedia. *Groupthink.* (2018). https://en.wikipedia.org/wiki/Groupthink.

46   Janis, I. L. "Groupthink." *Psychology Today* 5, 43–46, 74–76 (1972).

47   Lush, T. Scandals fester at unhealthy organizations, experts say. *Ithaca Journal* Aug 20, 2018.

48   Respondent's findings of fact, conclusions of law, argument and proposed order. Before Federal Trade Commission, Washington, DC. Docket No. 9175, 214 (New York: Bass & Ullman, 1985).

49   Potishman, N., McCulloch, C. E., Byers, T., Houghton, L., Nemoto, T., Graham, S. et al. Associations between breast cancer, triglycerides and cholesterol. *Nutrition and Cancer* 15, 205–215 (1991).

Chapter Six

1   Ansah, G. A., Chan, C. W., Touchburn, S. P., & Buckland, R. B. Selection for low yolk cholesterol in Leghorn-type chickens. *Poultry Sci.* 64, 1–5 (1985).

2   Ignatowski, A. Uber die Wirbung des tierischen eiweiss auf die aorta und die parenchymatosen organe der kaninchen. *Vrichows Arch. Pathol. Anat. Physiol. Klin. Med.* 198, 248–270 (1909).

3   Ignatowski, A. Influence de la nourriture animale sur l'organisme des papins. *Arch. Med. Exp. Anat. Pathol.* 210, 1–20 (1908).

4   Kritchevsky, D., in *Animal and vegetable proteins in lipid metabolism and atherosclerosis* (eds. M. J. Gibney & D. Kritchevsky), 1–8 (Alan R. Liss, 1983).

5   Kritchevsky, D. Dietary protein, cholesterol and atherosclerosis: a review of the early history. *J. Nutr.* 125, 589S–593S, doi:10.1093/jn/125.suppl_3.589S (1995).

6   Newburgh, L. H. & Clarkson, S. The production of arteriosclerosis in rabbits by feeding diets rich in meat. *Arch. Intern. Med.* 31, 653–676 (1923).

7   Newburgh, L. H. The production of Bright's disease by feeding high protein diets. *Arch. Intern. Med.* 24, 359–377 (1919).

8   Newburgh, L. H. & Clarkson, S. Production of atherosclerosis in rabbits by diet rich in animal protein. *JAMA* 79, 1106–1108 (1922).

9   Clarkson, S. & Newburgh, L. H. The relation between atherosclerosis and ingested cholesterol in the rabbit. *J. Exp. Med.* 43, 595–612 (1926).

10   Keys, A. The diet and the development of coronary heart disease. *J. Chronic Dis.* 4, 364–380 (1956).

11   Keys, A., Anderson, J. T., & Mickelsen, O. Serum cholesterol in men in basal and nonbasal states. *Science* 123, 29 (1956).

12   Campbell, T. C. Animal protein and ischemic heart disease. *Am. J. Clin. Nutr.* 71, 849–850 (2000).

13   Campbell, T. C. A plant based diet and animal protein: questioning dietary fat and considering animal protein as the main cause of heart disease. *J. Geriatric Cardiol.* 14, 331–337 (2017).

14   Carroll, K. K., in *Current topics in nutrition and disease, Vol. 8: Animal and vegetable proteins in lipid metabolism and atherosclerosis* (eds. M. J. Gibney & D. Kritchevsky), 9–18 (Alan R. Liss, 1983).

15   Gallagher, P. J. & Gibney, M. J., in *Current topics in nutrition and disease, Vol. 8: Animal and vegetable proteins in lipid metabolism and atherosclerosis* (eds. M. J. Gibney & D. Kritchevsky), 149–168 (Alan R. Liss, 1983).

16   Joop, M. A. v. R., Katan, M. B., & West, C. E., in *Current topics in nutrition and disease, Vol. 8: Animal and vegetable proteins in lipid metabolism and atherosclerosis* (eds. M. J. Gibney & D. Kritchevsky), 111–134 (Alan R. Liss, 1983).

17   Kim, D. N., Lee, K. T., Reiner, J. M., & Thomas, W. A., in *Current topics in nutrition and disease, Vol. 8: Animal and vegetable proteins in lipid metabolism and atherosclerosis* (eds. M. J. Gibney & D. Kritchevsky), 101–110 (Alan R. Liss, 1983).

18   Kritchevsky, D., Tepper, S. A., Czarnecki, S. K., Klurfeld, D. M., & Story, J. A., in *Current topics in nutrition and disease, Vol. 8: Animal and vegetable proteins in lipid metabolism and atherosclerosis* (eds. M. J. Gibney & D. Kritchevsky), 85–100 (Alan R. Liss, 1983).

19   Sirtori, C. R., Noseda, G., & Descovich, G. C., in *Current topics in nutrition and disease, Vol. 8: Animal and vegetable proteins in lipid metabolism and atherosclerosis* (eds. M. J. Gibney & D. Kritchevsky), 135–148 (Alan R. Liss, 1983).

20   Sugano, M., in *Current topics in nutrition and disease, Vol. 8: Animal and vegetable proteins in lipid metabolism and atherosclerosis* (eds. M. J. Gibney & D. Kritchevsky), 51–84 (Alan R. Liss, 1983).

21   Terpstra, A. H. M., Hermus, R. J. J., & West, C. E., in *Current topics in nutrition and disease, Vol. 8: Animal and vegetable proteins in lipid metabolism and atherosclerosis* (eds. M. J. Gibney & D. Kritchevsky), 19–49 (Alan R. Liss, 1983).

22   Gibney, M. J., & Kritchevsky, D., eds. *Current topics in nutrition and disease, Vol. 8: Animal and vegetable proteins in lipid metabolism and atherosclerosis* (Alan R. Liss, 1983).

23   Meeker, D. R. & Kesten, H. D. Experimental atherosclerosis and high protein diets. *Proc. Soc. Exp. Biol. Med.* 45, 543–545 (1940).

24   Meeker, D. R. & Kesten, H. D. Effect of high protein diets on experimental atherosclerosis of rabbits. *Arch. Pathology* 31, 147–162 (1941).

25   Kritchevsky, D., Tepper, S. A., Williams, D. E., & Story, J. A. Experimental atherosclerosis in rabbits fed cholesterol-free diets. Part 7. Interaction of animal or vegetable protein with fiber. *Atherosclerosis* 26, 397–403 (1977).

26   Terpstra, A. H., Harkes, L., & van der Veen, F. H. The effect of different proportions of casein in semipurified diets on the concentration of serum cholesterol and the lipoprotein composition in rabbits. *Lipids* 16, 114–119 (1981).

27   Sirtori, C. R., Noseda, G., & Descovich, G. C., in *Current topics in nutrition and disease, Vol. 8: Animal and vegetable proteins in lipid metabolism and atherosclerosis* (eds. M. J. Gibney & D. Kritchevsky), 135–148 (Alan R. Liss, 1983).

28   Descovich, G. C., Ceredi, C., Gaddi, A., Benassi, M. S., Mannino, G., Colombo, L. et al. Multicenter study of soybean protein diet for outpatient hypercholesterolemic patients. *Lancet* 2, 709–712 (1980).

29   Mitchell, H. H. A method of determining the biological value of protein. *J. Biol. Chem.* 58, 873–903 (1924).

30   Keys, A. Nutrition for the later years of life. *Public Health Rep* 67, 484–489 (1952).

31   Keys, A. Coronary heart disease in seven countries. *Circulation Suppl.* 41, I1–I211 (1970).

32   Keys, A. Coronary heart disease—the global picture. *Atherosclerosis* 22, 149–192 (1975).

33   US Department of Health and Human Services and US Department of Agriculture. *2015–2020 Dietary guidelines for Americans,* 8th ed. (Authors, 2015).

34   Keys, A. Diet and the epidemiology of coronary heart disease. *J. Am. Med. Assoc.* 164, 1912–1919 (1957).

35   Keys, A., in *Atherosclerosis and its origin* (eds. M. Sandler & G. H. Bourne), 263–299 (Academic Press, 1963).

36   Carroll, K. K., Braden, L. M., Bell, J. A., & Kalamegham, R. Fat and cancer. *Cancer* 58, 1818–1825 (1986).

37   American Heart Association. AHA Dietary Guidelines. Revision 2000: A statement for healthcare professionals from the Nutrition Committee of the American Heart Association. *Circulation* 102, 2296–2311 (2000).

38   O'Connor, T. P. & Campbell, T. C., in *Dietary fat and cancer* (eds. C. Ip, D. Birt, C. Mettlin, & A. Rogers), 731–771 (Alan R. Liss, 1986).

39   Committee on Diet, Nutrition, and Cancer. *Diet, nutrition and cancer.* (National Academies Press, 1982).

40   American Institute for Cancer Research and World Cancer Research Fund. *Food, nutrition and the prevention of cancer: a global perspective.* (Authors, 1997).

41   National Research Council & Committee on Diet and Health. *Diet and health: implications for reducing chronic disease risk.* (National Academies Press, 1989).

42   US Senate, Select Committee on Nutrition and Human Needs. *Dietary goals for the United States,* 2nd ed. (Washington, DC: US Government Printing Office, 1977), 83.

43   Armstrong, D. & Doll, R. Environmental factors and cancer incidence and mortality in different countries, with special reference to dietary practices. *Int. J. Cancer* 15, 617–631 (1975).

44   Willett, W. C., Hunter, D. J., Stampfer, M. J., Colditz, G., Manson, J. E., Spielgelman, D. et al. Dietary fat and fiber in relation to risk of breast cancer. An 8-year follow-up. *J. Am. Med. Assoc.* 268, 2037–2044 (1992).

45   Willett, W. C., Stampfer, M. J., Colditz, G. A., Rosner, B. A., Hennekens, C. H., & Speizer, F. E. Dietary fat and the risk of breast cancer. *New Engl. J. Med.* 316, 22–28 (1987).

46   Carroll, K. K. & Khor, H. T. Effects of dietary fat and dose level of 7,12 dimethylbenz(a)anthracene on mammary tumor incidence in rats. *Cancer Res.* 30, 2260–2264 (1970).

47   Gammal, E. B., Carroll, K. K., & Plunkett, E. R. Effects of dietary fat on mammary carciongenesis by 7,12-dimethylbenz(a)anthracene in rats. *Cancer Res.* 27, 1737–1742 (1967).

48   Hopkins, G. J. & Carroll, K. K. Relationship between amount and type of dietary fat in promotion of mammary carcinogenesis induced by 7, 12-dimethylbenzanthracene. *J Natl. Cancer Inst.* 62, 1009–1012 (1979).

49   Dias, C. B., Garg, R., Wood, L. G., & Garg, M. L. Saturated fat consumption may not be the main cause of increased blood lipid levels. *Med. Hypoth.* 82, 187–195 (2014).

50   Gershuni, V. M. Saturated fat: part of a healthy diet. *Curr. Nutr. Re.* 7, 85–96 (2018).

51   Sirtori, C. R., Gatti, E., Mantero, O., Conti, F., Agradi, E., Tremoli, E. et al. Clinical experience with the soybean protein diet in the treatment of hypercholesterolemia. *Am. J. Clin. Nutr.* 32, 1645–1658, doi:10.1093/ajcn/32.8.1645 (1979).

52   O'Connor, T. P., Roebuck, B. D., & Campbell, T. C. Dietary intervention during the post-dosing phase of L-azaserine-induced preneoplastic lesions. *J. Natl. Cancer Inst.* 75, 955–957 (1985).

53   O'Connor, T. P., Roebuck, B. D., Peterson, F., & Campbell, T. C. Effect of dietary intake of fish oil and fish protein on the development of L-azaserine-induced preneoplastic lesions in rat pancreas. *J. Natl. Cancer Inst.* 75, 959–962 (1985).

54   Abdelhamid, A. S., Brown, T. J., Brainard, J. S., Biswas, P., Thorpe, G. C., Moore, H. J. et al. Omega-3 fatty acids for the primary and secondary prevention of cardiovascular disease. *Cochrane Database Syst Rev* 11, CD003177, doi:10.1002/14651858.CD003177.pub4 (2018).

55   Simopoulos, A. P. An increase in the omega-6/omega-3 fatty acid ratio increases the risk for obesity. *Nutrients* 8, 128, doi:10.3390/nu8030128 (2016).

56   Simopoulos, A. P. & DiNicolantonio, J. J. The importance of a balanced omega-6 to omega-3 ratio in the prevention and management of obesity. *Open Heart* 3, e000385, doi:10.1136/openhrt-2015-000385 (2016).

57   Ponnampalam, E. N., Mann, N. J., & Sinclair, A. J. Effect of feeding systems on omega-3 fatty acids, conjugated linoleic acid and trans fatty acids in Australian beef cuts: potential impact on human health. *Asia Pac. J. Clin. Nutr.* 15, 21–29 (2006).

58   Grosso, G., Yang, J., Marventano, S., Micek, A., Galvano, F., & Kales, S. N. Nut consumption on all-cause, cardiovascular, and cancer mortality risk: a systematic review and meta-analysis of epidemiologic studies. *Am. J. Clin. Nutr.* 101, 783–793, doi:10.3945/ajcn.114.099515 (2015).

59   Schwingshackl, L., Hoffman, G., Missbach, B., Stelmach-Mardas, M., & Boeing, H. An umbrella review of nuts intake and risk of cardiovascular disease. *Current Pharm. Design* 23, 1016–1027 (2017).

60   Keys, A. *Seven countries. A multivariate analysis of death and coronary heart disease.* (Harvard University Press, 1980).

61   Kromhout, D., Menotti, A., Bloemberg, B., Aravanis, C., Blackburn, H., Buzina, R. et al. Dietary saturated and trans fatty acids and cholesterol and 25-year mortality from coronary heart disease: the Seven Countries Study. *Prev. Med.* 24, 308–315 (1995).

62   McGee, D. L., Reed, D. M. & Yano, K. Ten-year incidence of coronary heart disease in the Honolulu Heart Program: relationship to nutrient intake. *Am. J. Epidemiol.* 119, 667–676 (1984).

63   Kromhout, D. & Coulander, C. L. Diet, prevalence and 10 year mortality from coronary heart disease in 871 middle-aged men. *Am. J. Epidemiol.* 119, 733–741 (1984).

64   Garcia-Palmieri, M. R., Sorlie, P., Tillotson, J., Costas, R. Jr., Cordero, E., & Rodriguez, M. Relationship of dietary intake to subsequent coronary heart disease incidence: the Puerto Rican Heart Health Program. *Am. J. Clin. Nutr.* 33, 1818–1827 (1980).

65   Morris, J. N., Marr, J. W., & Clayton, O. B. Diet and heart: a postscript. *Brit. Med. J.* 2, 1307–1314 (1977).

66   Hu, F. B., Stampfer, M. J., Manson, J. E., Rimm, E., Colditz, G. A., Rosner, B. A. et al. Dietary fat intake and the risk of coronary heart disease in women. *New Engl. J. Med.* 337, 1491–1499, doi:10.1056/NEJM199711203372102 (1997).

67   Hu, F. B., Manson, J. E., & Willett, W. C. Types of dietary fat and risk of coronary heart disease: a critical review. *J. Am. Coll. Nutr.* 20, 5–19 (2001).

68   Youngman, L. D., Park, J. Y., & Ames, B. N. Protein oxidation associated with aging is reduced by dietary restriction of protein or calories. *Proc. National Acad. Sci.* 89, 9112–9116 (1992).

69   De, A. K., Chipalkatti, S., & Aiyar, A. S. Some biochemical parameters of ageing in relation to dietary protein. *Mech Ageing Dev* 21, 37–48 (1983).

70   Sanz, A., Caro, P., & Barja, G. Protein restriction without strong caloric restriction decreases mitochondrial oxygen radical production and oxidative DNA damage in rat liver. *J. Bioenergetics Biomembranes* 36, 545–552 (2004).

71   Huang, H. H., Hawrylewicz, E. J., Kissane, J. Q., & Drab, E. A. Effect of protein diet on release of prolactin and ovarian steroids in female rats. *Nutrition Reports International* 26, 807–820 (1982).

72   Asao, T., Abdel-Kader, M. M., Chang, S. B., Wick, E. L., & Wogan, G. N. Aflatoxins B and G. *J. Am. Chem. Soc.* 85, 1706–1707 (1963).

73   Wogan, G. N., & Newberne, P. M. Dose-response characteristics of aflatoxin B_1 carcinogenesis in the rat. *Cancer Res.* 27, 2370–2376 (1967).

74   Ayres, J. L., Lee, D. J., Wales, J. H., & Sinnhuber, R. O. Aflatoxin structure and hepatocarcinogenicity in rainbow trout. *J. Natl. Cancer Inst.* 46, 561–564 (1971).

75   Campbell, T. C., Sinnhuber, R. O., Lee, D. J., Wales, J. H., & Salamat, L. A. Brief communication: hepatocarcinogenic material in urine specimens from humans consuming aflatoxin. *J. Nat. Cancer Inst.* 52, 1647–1649 (1974).

76   Campbell, T. C. & Hayes, J. R. The role of aflatoxin in its toxic lesion. *Tox. Appl. Pharm.* 35, 199–222 (1976).

77   Campbell, T. C. Present day knowledge on aflatoxin. *Philadelphia Journal of Nutrition* 20, 193–201 (1967).

78   Campbell, T. C., Caedo, J. P., Jr., Bulatao-Jayme, J., Salamat, L., & Engel, R. W. Aflatoxin M_1 in human urine. *Nature* 227, 403–404 (1970).

79   Campbell, T. C. Chemical carcinogens and human risk assessment. *Fed. Proc.* 39, 2467–2484 (1980).

80   Campbell, T. C., & Hayes, J. R. Role of nutrition in the drug metabolizing system. *Pharmacol. Revs.* 26, 171–197 (1974).

81   Hayes, J. R., & Campbell, T. C., in *Modifiers of chemical carcinogenesis* (ed. T. J. Slaga), 207–241 (Raven Press, 1980).

82   Chen, J., Campbell, T. C., Li, J., & Peto, R. *Diet, life-style and mortality in China. A study of the characteristics of 65 Chinese counties.* (Oxford University Press; Cornell University Press; People's Medical Publishing House, 1990).

83   Campbell, T. C., Chen, J., Liu, C., Li, J., & Parpia, B. Non-association of aflatoxin with primary liver cancer in a cross-sectional ecologic survey in the People's Republic of China. *Cancer Res.* 50, 6882–6893 (1990).

84   Campbell, T. C. Nutrition renaissance and public health policy. *J. Nutr. Biology* 3, 124–138, doi:10.1080/01635581.2017.1339094 (2017).

85   Campbell, T. C. Cancer prevention and treatment by wholistic nutrition. *J. Nat. Sci.* Oct 3, e448 (2017).

86   Weisburger, E. K. History of the bioassay program of the National Cancer Institute. *Prog. Exp. Tumor Res.* 26, 187–201 (1983).

87   International Agency for Cancer Research. Press release: IARC monographs evaluate consumption of red meat and processed meat. (2015).

88   Wikipedia. *Carcinogen.* https://en.wikipedia.org/wiki/Carcinogen (2020).

89   National Toxicology Program. *Report on carcinogens*. 499 (2011).

90   National Toxicology Program. *Ninth report on carcinogens* (rev. January 2001).

91   National Toxicology Program. https://ntp.niehs.nih.gov/.

92   Huff, J. Long-term chemical carcinogenesis bioassays predict human cancer hazards. Issues, controversies, and uncertainties. *Ann. NY Acad. Sci.* 895, 56–79 (1999).

93   Huff, J., Jacobson, M. F., & Davis, D. L. The limits of two-year bioassay exposure regimens for identifying chemical carcinogens. *Environ. Health Perspect.* 116, 1439–1442 (2008).

94   National Toxicology Program. *14th Report on Carcinogens*, Process and Listing Criteria. (November 3, 2016). https://ntp.niehs.nih.gov/pubhealth/roc/process/index.html.

95   Knight, A., Bailey, J., & Balcombe, J. Animal carcinogenicity studies: 3. Alternatives to the bioassay. *Altern. Lab. Anim.* 34, 39–48 (2006).

96   Knight, A., Bailey, J., & Balcombe, J. Animal carcinogenicity studies: 2. Obstacles to extrapolation of data to humans. *Altern. Lab. Anim.* 34, 29–38 (2006).

97   Knight, A., Bailey, J., & Balcombe, J. Animal carcinogenicity studies: 1. Poor human predictivity. *Altern. Lab. Anim.* 34, 19–27 (2006).

98   Wikipedia. *Human genome project.* https://en.wikipedia.org/wiki/Human_Genome_Project (2018).

99   National Cancer Institute. What is cancer? (Updated February 9, 2015). http://www.cancer.gov/about-cancer/what-is-cancer.

100   Appleton, B. S., Goetchius, M. P., & Campbell, T. C. Linear dose-response curve for the hepatic macromolecular binding of aflatoxin B_1 in rats at very low exposures. *Cancer Res.* 42, 3659–3662 (1982).

101   Dunaif, G. E. & Campbell, T. C. Dietary protein level and aflatoxin B1-induced preneoplastic hepatic lesions in the rat. *J. Nutr.* 117, 1298–1302 (1987).

102   Dunaif, G. E. & Campbell, T. C. Relative contribution of dietary protein level and aflatoxin B_1 dose in generation of presumptive preneoplastic foci in rat liver. *J. Natl. Cancer Inst.* 78, 365–369 (1987).

103   Schulsinger, D. A., Root, M. M., & Campbell, T. C. Effect of dietary protein quality on development of aflatoxin B_1-induced hepatic preneoplastic lesions. *J. Natl. Cancer Inst.* 81, 1241–1245 (1989).

104   Berwyn, B. IPCC: radical energy transformation needed to avoid 1.5 degrees global warming. *Inside Climate News* (2018). https://insideclimatenews.org/news/07102018/ipcc-climate-change-science-report-data-carbon-emissions-heat-waves-extreme-weather-oil-gas-agriculture.

105   Strona, G. & Bradshaw, C. J. A. Co-extinctions annihilate planetary life during extreme environmental change. *Sci. Rpts.* 8, doi:10.1038/s41598-018-35068-1 (2018).

106   MacFarlane, D. All the species that went extinct in 2018, and ones on the brink for 2019. *Environment* (2019). https://weather.com/science/environment/news/2019-01-02-extinct-animal-species-2018.

107   Sanchez-Bayo, F. & Wyckhuys, K. A. G. Worldwide decline of the entofauna: a review of its drivers. *Biolological Conservation* 232, 8–27 (2016).

108   Goodland, R. & Anhang, J. Livestock and climate change. *World Watch*, 1–10 (2009).

109   Brown, L. R. *Tough choices: facing the challenge of food scarcity.* (W. W. Norton & Company, 1996).

110   Hindhede, M. The biological value of bread-protein. *Biochem. J.* 20, 330–334 (1926).

111   Bridi, D., Altenhofen, S., Gonzalez, J. B., Reolon, G. K., & Bonan, C. D. Glyphosate and Roundup® alter morphology and behavior in zebrafish. *Toxicology* 392, 32–39, doi:10.1016/j.tox.2017.10.007 (2017).

112   United Nations, Food and Agriculture Organization. *Livestock's long shadow: environmental issues and options.* (Food and Agriculture Organization, 2006).

113   Compassion in World Farming. *Strategic plan 2013–2017.* https://www.ciwf.org.uk/media/3640540/ciwf_strategic_plan_20132017.pdf.

114   Oppenlander, R. *Food choice and sustainability.* (Minneapolis: Langdon Street Press, 2013), 46.

115 Hatchett, A. N. Bovines and global warming: how the cows are heating things up and what can be done to cool them down. *William & Mary Environmental Law and Policy Review* 29, 767–780 (2005).

Chapter Seven

1   Gibney, M. J. & Kritchevsky, D., eds. *Current topics in nutrition and disease, Vol. 8: Animal and vegetable proteins in lipid metabolism and atherosclerosis* (Alan R. Liss, 1983).
2   Hill, A. B. The environment and disease: association or causation? *Proc. Royal Soc. Med.* 108, 32–37 (1965).

Chapter Eight

1   Committee on Diet, Nutrition, and Cancer. *Diet, Nutrition and Cancer.* (National Academies Press, 1982).
2   National Research Council and Institute of Medicine, Committee on Diet and Health. *Diet and Health: Implications for Reducing Chronic Disease Risk.* (National Academy Press, 1989.)
3   US Department of Agriculture. *FoodData Central* (2020). https://fdc.nal.usda.gov/.
4   Reboul, E., Thap, S., Perrot, E., Amiot, M. J., Lairon, D., & Borel, P. Effect of the main dietary antioxidants (carotenoids, gamma-tocopherol, polyphenols, and vitamin C) on alpha-tocopherol absorption. *European Journal of Clinical Nutrition* 61, 1167–1173, doi:10.1038/sj.ejcn.1602635 (2007).
5   Campbell, T. C. Energy balance: interpretation of data from rural China. *Toxicological Sciences* 52, 87–94 (1999).
6   Ornish, D. *Eat more, weigh less.* (HarperCollins Publishers, Inc., 1993).
7   Shintani, T. *Dr. Shintani's eat more, weigh less diet.* (Halpax Publishing, 1993).
8   Russell, R. National Weight Control Registry. Last modified 2020. https://en.wikipedia.org/wiki/National_Weight_Control_Registry.
9   Swann, J. P. The history of efforts to regulate dietary supplement in the USA. *Drug Testing Analysis* 8, 271–282 (2015).
10   Cision PR Newswire. *Dietary supplements market to reach USD 216.3 billion by 2026. Reports and Data.* https://www.prnewswire.com/news-releases/dietary-supplements-market-to-reach-usd-216-3-billion-by-2026--reports-and-data-300969115.html (December 4, 2019).
11   Dietary Supplement Health and Education Act of 1994. Pub. L. No. 103-417, 108 Stat. 4325.
12   US Food and Drug Administration. *Dietary supplement health and education act of 1994,* http://vm.cfsan.fda.gov/~dms/dietsupp.html (1995) (site discontinued).
13   Respondent's findings of fact, conclusions of law, argument and proposed order. Before Federal Trade Commission, Washington, DC. Docket No. 9175, 214 (New York: Bass & Ullman, 1985).
14   Omenn, G. S., Goodman, G. E., Thornquist, M. D., Balmes, J., Cullen, M. R., Glass, A. et al. Risk factors for lung cancer and for intervention effects in CARET, the Beta-Carotene and Retinol Efficacy Trial. *J. Natl. Cancer Inst.* 88, 1550–1559 (1996).
15   Kelloff, G. J., Crowell, J. A., Hawk, E. T., Steele, V. E., Lubet, R. A., Boone, C. W. et al. Strategy and planning for chemopreventive drug development: clinical development plans II. *J. Cell. Biochem.* 26S, 54–315 (1996).
16   US Preventive Services Task Force. Routine vitamin supplementation to prevent cancer and cardiovascular disease: recommendations and rationale. *Ann. Internal Med.* 139, 51–55 (2003).
17   Omenn, G. S., Goodman, G. E., Thornquist, M. D., Balmes, J., Cullen, M. R., Glass, A. et al. Effects of a combination of beta carotene and vitamin A on lung cancer and cardiovascular disease. *New Engl. J. Med.* 334, 1150–1155 (1996).
18   Peto, R., Doll, R., & Buckley, J. D. Can dietary beta-carotene materially reduce human cancer rates? *Nature* 290, 201–208 (1981).
19   Shekelle, R. B. & Raynor, W. J., Jr. Dietary vitamin A and risk of cancer in the Western Electric Study. *Lancet* 2, 1185–1190 (1981).

20   Morris, C. D. & Carson, S. Routine vitamin supplementation to prevent cardiovascular disease: a summary of the evidence for the U.S. Preventive Services Task Force. *Ann. Internal Med.* 139, 56–70 (2003).

21   Goodman, B. Experts: don't waste your money on multivitamins. *WebMD Health Newsletter* (2013). https://www.webmd.com/vitamins-and-supplements/news/20131216/experts-dont-waste-your-money-on-multivitamins#1.

22   ScienceDaily. Most popular vitamin and mineral supplements provide no health benefit, study finds. *Science News* (2018). https://www.sciencedaily.com/releases/2018/05/180528171511.htm.

23   IBISWorld. Vitamin & Supplement Manufacturing—US Market Research Report. (2018). https://www.ibisworld.com/industry-trends/market-research-reports/manufacturing/chemical/vitamin-supplement-manufacturing.html.

24   Grand View Research. Dietary supplements market size worth $278.02 billion by 2024. (2018). https://www.grandviewresearch.com/industry-analysis/dietary-supplements-market.

25   United States Department of Health and Human Services. *The Surgeon General's Report on Nutrition and Health.* (Superintendent of Documents, US Government Printing Office, 1988).

26   National Research Council & Committee on Diet and Health. *Diet and health: implications for reducing chronic disease risk.* (National Academies Press, 1989).

27   American Institute for Cancer Research and World Cancer Research Fund. *Food, nutrition and the prevention of cancer: a global perspective.* (Authors, 1997).

Chapter Nine

1   Carroll, K. K., Braden, L. M., Bell, J. A., & Kalamegham, R. Fat and cancer. *Cancer* 58, 1818–1825 (1986).

2   National Research Council & Committee on Diet and Health. *Diet and health: implications for reducing chronic disease risk.* (National Academies Press, 1989).

3   Campbell, T. C. A plant based diet and animal protein: questioning dietary fat and considering animal protein as the main cause of heart disease. *J. Geriatric Cardiol.* 14, 331–337 (2017).

4   Armstrong, D. & Doll, R. Environmental factors and cancer incidence and mortality in different countries, with special reference to dietary practices. *Int. J. Cancer* 15, 617–631 (1975).

5   Newburgh, L. H. & Clarkson, S. The production of arteriosclerosis in rabbits by feeding diets rich in meat. *Arch. Intern. Med.* 31, 653–676 (1923).

6   Ganmaa, D. & Sato, A. The possible role of female sex hormones in milk from pregnant cows in the development of breast, ovarian and corpus uteri cancers. *Med. Hypotheses* 65, 1028–1037, doi:10.1016/j.mehy.2005.06.026 (2005).

7   Connor, W. E. & Connor, S. L. The key role of nutritional factors in the prevention of coronary heart disease. *Prev. Med.* 1, 49–83 (1972).

8   Jolliffe, N. & Archer, M. Statistical associations between international coronary heart disease death rates and certain environmental factors. *J. Chronic Dis.* 9, 636–652 (1959).

9   Campbell, T. M. I. & Campbell, T. C. The breadth of evidence favoring a whole-foods, plant-based diet. Part II, malignancy and inflammatory diseases. *Primary Care Reports* 18, 25–35 (2012).

10   World Cancer Research Fund/American Institute for Cancer Research. *Food, nutrition, physical activity, and prevention of cancer: a global perspective.* (American Institute for Cancer Research, 2007), 517.

11   Hildenbrand, G. L. G., Hildenbrand, L. C., Bradford, K., & Cavin, S. W. Five-year survival rates of melanoma patients treated by diet therapy after the manner of Gerson: a retrospective review. *Alternative Therapies in Health and Medicine* 1, 29–37 (1995).

12   Morrison, L. M. Arteriosclerosis. *JAMA* 145, 1232–1236 (1951).

13   Morrison, L. M. Diet in coronary atherosclerosis. *JAMA* 173, 884–888 (1960).

14   Steinberg, D. Thematic review series: the pathogenesis of atherosclerosis: an interpretive history of the cholesterol controversy, part III: mechanistically defining the role of hyperlipidemia. *J. Lipid Res.* 46, 2037–2051, doi:10.1194/jlr.R500010-JLR200 (2005).

15   Ornish, D., Brown, S. E., Scherwitz, L. W., Billings, J. H., Armstrong, W. T., Ports, T. A. et al. Can lifestyle changes reverse coronary heart disease? *Lancet* 336, 129–133 (1990).

16   Esselstyn, C. B., Jr. Updating a 12-year experience with arrest and reversal therapy for coronary heart disease (an overdue requiem for palliative cardiology). *Am. J. Cardiol.* 84, 339–341 (1999).

17   Esselstyn, C. B., Ellis, S. G., Medendorp, S. V., & Crowe, T. D. A strategy to arrest and reverse coronary artery disease: a 5-year longitudinal study of a single physician's practice. *J. Family Practice* 41, 560–568 (1995).

18   Esselstyn, C. B. J., Gendy, G., Doyle, J., Golubic, M., & Roizen, M. F. A way to reverse CAD? *J. Fam. Pract.* 63, 356–364b (2014).

19   Campbell, T. C. Present day knowledge on aflatoxin. *Philadelphia Journal of Nutrition* 20, 193–201 (1967).

20   Campbell, T. C., Caedo, J. P., Jr., Bulatao-Jayme, J., Salamat, L., & Engel, R. W. Aflatoxin M_1 in human urine. *Nature* 227, 403–404 (1970).

21   Lancaster, M. C., Jenkins, F. P., & Philp, J. M. Toxicity associated with certain samples of ground-nuts. *Nature* 192, 1095–1096 (1961).

22   Wogan, G. N., in *Methods in cancer research*, Vol. 7 (ed. H. Busch), 309–344 (Academic Press, 1973).

23   Madhavan, T. V. & Gopalan, C. The effect of dietary protein on carcinogenesis of aflatoxin. *Arch. Path.* 85, 133–137 (1968).

24   Schulsinger, D. A., Root, M. M., & Campbell, T. C. Effect of dietary protein quality on development of aflatoxin B_1-induced hepatic preneoplastic lesions. *J. Natl. Cancer Inst.* 81, 1241–1245 (1989).

25   Youngman, L. D. & Campbell, T. C. Inhibition of aflatoxin B_1-induced gamma-glutamyl transpeptidase positive (GGT+) hepatic preneoplastic foci and tumors by low protein diets: evidence that altered GGT+ foci indicate neoplastic potential. *Carcinogenesis* 13, 1607–1613 (1992).

26   Gurtoo, H. L. & Campbell, T. C. A kinetic approach to a study of the induction of rat liver microsomal hydroxylase after pretreatment with 3,4-benzpyrene and aflatoxin B_1. *Biochem. Pharmacol.* 19, 1729–1735 (1970).

27   Nerurkar, L. S., Hayes, J. R., & Campbell, T. C. The reconstitution of hepatic microsomal mixed function oxidase activity with fractions derived from weanling rats fed different levels of protein. *J. Nutr.* 108, 678–686 (1978).

28   Preston, R. S., Hayes, J. R., & Campbell, T. C. The effect of protein deficiency on the in vivo binding of aflatoxin B_1 to rat liver macromolecules. *Life Sci.* 19, 1191–1198 (1976).

29   Prince, L. O. & Campbell, T. C. Effects of sex difference and dietary protein level on the binding of aflatoxin B_1 to rat liver chromatin proteins in vivo. *Cancer Res.* 42, 5053–5059 (1982).

30   Krieger, E. *Increased voluntary exercise by Fisher 344 rats fed low protein diets* (undergraduate thesis, Cornell University, 1988).

31   Krieger, E., Youngman, L. D., & Campbell, T. C. The modulation of aflatoxin (AFB_1) induced preneoplastic lesions by dietary protein and voluntary exercise in Fischer 344 rats. *FASEB J.* 2, 3304 Abs. (1988).

32   Horio, F., Youngman, L. D., Bell, R. C., & Campbell, T. C. Thermogenesis, low-protein diets, and decreased development of AFB_1-induced preneoplastic foci in rat liver. *Nutrition and Cancer* 16, 31–41 (1991).

33   Youngman, L. D., Park, J. Y., & Ames, B. N. Protein oxidation associated with aging is reduced by dietary restriction of protein or calories. *Proc. National Acad. Sci.* 89, 9112–9116 (1992).

34   Chen, J., Campbell, T. C., Li, J., & Peto, R. *Diet, life-style and mortality in China. A study of the characteristics of 65 Chinese counties.* (Oxford University Press; Cornell University Press; People's Medical Publishing House, 1990).

35   Centers for Disease Control and Prevention. *Heart disease.* (2020). https://www.cdc.gov/nchs/fastats/heart-disease.htm.

36   Campbell, T. C., Chen, J., Brun, T., Parpia, B., Qu, Y., Chen, C. et al. China: from diseases of poverty to diseases of affluence. Policy implications of the epidemiological transition. *Ecology of Food and Nutrition* 27, 133–144 (1992).

37   Kannel, W. B., Neaton, J. D., Wentworth, D., Thomas, H. E., Stamler, J., Hulley, S. B. et al. Overall and coronary heart disease mortality rates in relation to major risk factors in 325,348 men screened for the MRFIT. Multiple Risk Factor Intervention Trial. *Am. Heart J.* 112, 825–836 (1986).

Chapter Ten

1   Campbell, T. C. & Campbell, T. M., II. *The China Study: startling implications for diet, weight loss, and long-term health.* (BenBella Books, Inc., 2005), 417.

2   Campbell, T. C., Chen, J., Liu, C., Li, J., & Parpia, B. Non-association of aflatoxin with primary liver cancer in a cross-sectional ecologic survey in the People's Republic of China. *Cancer Res.* 50, 6882–6893 (1990).

3   Hu, J., Chisari, F. V., & Campbell, T. C. Modulating effect of dietary protein on transgene expression in hepatitis B virus (HBV) transgenic mice. *Cancer Research* 35, 104Abs (1994).

4   Prince, L. O. & Campbell, T. C. Effects of sex difference and dietary protein level on the binding of aflatoxin B_1 to rat liver chromatin proteins in vivo. *Cancer Res.* 42, 5053–5059 (1982).

5   Appleton, B. S. & Campbell, T. C. Effect of high and low dietary protein on the dosing and post-dosing periods of aflatoxin B_1-induced hepatic preneoplastic lesion development in the rat. *Cancer Res.* 43, 2150–2154 (1983).

6   Chen, J., Campbell, T. C., Li, J., & Peto, R. *Diet, life-style and mortality in China. A study of the characteristics of 65 Chinese counties.* (Oxford University Press; Cornell University Press; People's Medical Publishing House, 1990).

7   American Institute for Cancer Research and World Cancer Research Fund. *Food, nutrition and the prevention of cancer: a global perspective.* (Authors, 1997).

8   American Association of University Professors. Reports and publications: 1940 statement of principles on academic freedom and tenure. https://www.aaup.org/report/1940-statement-principles -academic-freedom-and-tenure.

9   Liu, M. & Mallon, W. T. Tenure in transition: trends in basic science faculty appointment policies at U.S. medical schools. *Acad. Med.* 79, 205–213 (2004).

10   Barakat, M. Documents show ties between university, conservative donors. (2018). https://www .usnews.com/news/best-states/virginia/articles/2018-04-30/documents-show-ties-between -university-conservative-donors.

11   Green, E. L. & Saul, S. What Charles Koch and other donors to George Mason University got for their money. *New York Times* (2018). https://www.nytimes.com/2018/05/05/us/koch-donors -george-mason.html.

12   US Department of Health and Human Services and US Department of Agriculture. *2015–2020 dietary guidelines for Americans,* 8th ed. (Authors, 2015).

13   Campbell, T. C. Dr. Campbell's recommended dietary guidelines. *T. Colin Campbell Center for Nutrition Studies* (2015). https://nutritionstudies.org/2015-dietary-guidelines-commentary/.

14   Kirkey, S. Got milk? Not so much. Health Canada's new food guide drops "milk and alternatives" and favours plant-based protein. *National Post* (2019). https://nationalpost.com/health/health -canada-new-food-guide-2019.

15   Gulshan, V., Peng, L., Coram, M., Stumpe, M. C., Wu, D., Narayanaswamy, A. et al. Development and validation of a deep learning algorithm for detection of diabetic retinopathy in retinal fundus photographs. *JAMA* 316, 2402–2410, doi:10.1001/jama.2016.17216 (2016).

16   Esteva, A., Kuprel, B., Novoa, R. A., Ko, J., Swetter, S. M., Blau, H. M. et al. Dermatologist-level classification of skin cancer with deep neural networks. *Nature* 542, 115–118, doi:10.1038/ nature21056 (2017).

17   Rajpurkar, M., Biss, T., Amankwah, E. K., Martinez, D., Williams, S., Van Ommen, C. H. et al. Pulmonary embolism and in situ pulmonary artery thrombosis in paediatrics. A systematic review. *Thromb. Haemost.* 117, 1199–1207, doi:10.1160/TH16-07-0529 (2017).

Postscript

1   Chen, J., Campbell, T. C., Li, J., & Peto, R. *Diet, life-style and mortality in China. A study of the characteristics of 65 Chinese counties.* (Oxford University Press; Cornell University Press; People's Medical Publishing House, 1990).

2   Chen, J., Peto, R., Pan, W., Liu, B., & Campbell, T. C. *Mortality, biochemistry, diet and lifestyle in rural China. Geographic study of the characteristics of 69 counties in mainland China and 16 areas in Taiwan.* (Oxford University Press, 2006).

3   Hu, J., Cheng, Z., Chisari, F. V., Vu, T. H., Hoffman, A. R., & Campbell, T. C. Repression of hepatitis B virus (HBV) transgene and HBV-induced liver injury by low protein diet. *Oncogene* **15**, 2795–2801 (1997).

4   Cheng, Z., Hu, J., King, J., Jay, G., & Campbell, T. C. Inhibition of hepatocellular carcinoma development in hepatitis B virus transfected mice by low dietary casein. *Hepatology* **26**, 1351–1354 (1997).

5   Hu, J., Chisari, F. V., & Campbell, T. C. Modulating effect of dietary protein on transgene expression in hepatitis B virus (HBV) transgenic mice. *Cancer Research* **35**, 104Abs (1994).

6   Gelles, D. & Drucker, J. Corporate insiders pocket $1 billion in rush for coronavirus vaccine. (2020). https://www.nytimes.com/2020/07/25/business/coronavirus-vaccine-profits-vaxart.html.

Afterword

1   Kagan, J. European Medicines Agency (EMA). *Investopedia* (2019). https://www.investopedia.com/terms/e/european-medicines-agency-ema.asp.

2   Morgan, G., Ward, R., & Barton, M. The contribution of cytotoxic chemotherapy to 5-year survival in adult malignancies. *Clin. Oncol. (R. Coll. Radiol.)* 16, 549–560 (2004).

3   Scheiber, N. Why Wendy's is facing campus protests (it's about the tomatoes). *New York Times,* March 7, 2019, https://www.nytimes.com/2019/03/07/business/economy/wendys-farm-workers-tomatoes.html; Boycott Wendy's homepage, http://www.boycott-wendys.org/.

INDEX

ABOUT THE AUTHORS

For more than fifty years, **Dr. T. Colin Campbell** has been at the forefront of nutrition research. His legacy, the China Study, was, at that time, the most comprehensive study of health and nutrition ever conducted. Dr. Campbell is Jacob Gould Schurman Professor Emeritus of Nutritional Biochemistry at Cornell University. He has received more than seventy grant-years of peer-reviewed research funding and authored more than 350 research papers, most being peer-reviewed. The China Study was the culmination of a twenty-year partnership of Cornell University, Oxford University, and the Chinese Academy of Preventative Medicine. In 1997, it was cited by the Chinese Ministry of Health as the most important study in medicine in China for the 20-yeriod 1978–1997. He also has been a member of several expert panels on food, nutrition and health, especially those of the U.S. National Academy of Sciences and the U.S. National Institutes of Health (NIH). He has been the recipient of three lifetime achievement awards.

Nelson Disla lives in Carrboro, North Carolina. He is a graduate of the University of North Carolina at Chapel Hill, where he studied English. He works as a writer and editor.

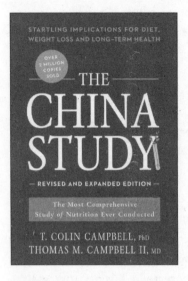
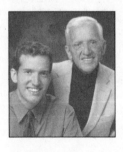

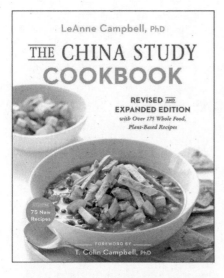
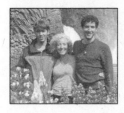

From the author of the groundbreaking bestseller,
The China Study, comes the much-anticipated . . .

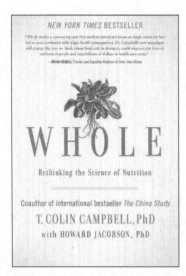

NEW YORK TIMES BESTSELLER

"Whole makes a convincing case that modern nutrition's focus on single nutrients has led to mass confusion with tragic health consequences. Dr. Campbell's new paradigm will change the way we think about food and, in doing so, could improve the lives of millions of people and save billions of dollars in health care costs."

—BRIAN WENDEL, Creator and Executive Producer of *Forks Over Knives*

WHOLE

Rethinking the Science of Nutrition

Coauthor of international bestseller *The China Study*

T. COLIN CAMPBELL, PhD

with HOWARD JACOBSON, PhD

Whole

Rethinking the Science of Nutrition

By T. COLIN CAMPBELL, PhD
and HOWARD JACOBSON, PhD

Whole picks up where The China Study left off. The China Study revealed what we should eat and provided the powerful empirical support for this answer. Whole answers why a whole-food, plant-based diet provides optimal nutrition. Whole demonstrates how far the scientific reductionism of the nutrition orthodoxy has gotten off track and reveals the elegant holistic workings of nutrition, from the cellular level to the operation of the entire organism. Whole is a marvelous journey through cutting-edge thinking on nutrition, led by one of the masters of the science.

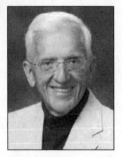

For more than 40 years, T. COLIN CAMPBELL, PhD, has been at the forefront of nutrition research. His legacy, the China Study, is the most comprehensive study of health and nutrition ever conducted. Dr. Campbell is the Jacob Gould Schurman Professor Emeritus of Nutritional Biochemistry at Cornell University. He has received more than 70 grant-years of peer-reviewed research funding and authored more than 300 research papers. The China Study was the culmination of a 20-year partnership of Cornell University, Oxford University, and the Chinese Academy of Preventive Medicine.

Visit **THECHINASTUDY.COM** to learn more!